Manual Thermal Diagnosis

Manual Thermal Diagnosis

By Jean-Pierre-Barral

Illustrated by Jacques Roth

Eastland Press
SEATTLE

Originally published as *Diagnostic Thermique Manuel*, Maloine (Paris), 1994.

English language edition © 1996 by Eastland Press, Incorporated
P.O. Box 12689, Seattle, Washington 98111
All rights reserved.

No part of this book may be reproduced, stored in a retrieval system, or transmitted in any form or by any means without the prior written permission of the publisher.

Library of Congress Catalog Card Number: 94-61966
International Standard Book Number: 0-939616-24-6
Printed in the United States of America.

English translation by John Blankenship and Dan Bensky, D.O.
English language edition edited by Stephen Anderson, Ph.D.
    and Dan Bensky, D.O.
Book design by Gordon Frazier

2 4 6 8 10 9 7 5 3

Contents

I. Introduction 1
II. Heat and Infrared 5
III. Body Temperature 11
IV. Skin Temperature 19
V. Thermal Control and Regulation 29
VI. Manual Thermal Diagnosis 37
VII. Cranium, Face, and Neck 55
VIII. Thorax 69
IX. Abdomen 85
X. Pelvis 99
XI. Posterior Visceral Projections: Osteoarticular System ... 105
XII. Afterword 115

Appendix: Psychological, Emotional,
and Behavioral Correspondences of the Organs 117
Bibliography 123
Index 131

CHAPTER 1

Introduction

IN MANUAL thermal diagnosis, the hands are held near but not touching the patient's skin in order to sense variations in thermal radiation from the body. These variations permit the localization and interpretation of pathological zones.

This phenomenon has been recognized for thousands of years. Dr. Bruno Roche (Geneva, Switzerland) attributes the earliest known thermal diagnosis to Hippocrates. He is said to have covered patients with mud, noted the places where the mud dried most rapidly, and found that these were typically sites of medical problems.

Animal and human thermosensitivity

Highly sensitive thermoreceptors are found in many animal species.

Rattlesnakes, like other pit vipers, have a specialized sensory organ in a pit located below the eye. The receptors in the organ are very sensitive to temperature variation, and can respond to differences as small as 0.003°C. This is equivalent to a stimulation threshold of 5–10 calories in 0.1 second! The rattlesnake can therefore sense the location of a warm-blooded animal (e.g. mouse) in total darkness, without using visual or auditory cues. Studies have shown that a blind rattlesnake can guide itself with precision toward a warm object.

Potential sensory acuity in humans is far greater than most people realize. The conditions of modern civilization discourage most of us from reaching this potential. A wine connoisseur can identify the geographic origin and year of a wine simply by tasting it. Yet chemical analysis of the wine does not reveal the qualities which make such precision possible.

The sensitivity of the human hand to pressure, motion, and heat is extremely high. Unfortunately, in modern medicine, manual diagnostic techniques have steadily given way to batteries of laboratory tests requiring sophisticated and expensive machines. These tests are often invasive. I do not dispute the utility of these tests. However, I do regret the modern tendency to use them unnecessarily in simple cases, and the fact that their use discourages practitioners from using their hands.

My introduction to manual thermal diagnosis

In 1970, I casually gestured with my hand in the process of requesting a female patient to change position on the examining table. I was surprised to feel a sensation of heat over the patient's thorax with my hand, and asked if there had been any problems in that area. She reported a breast tumor which had been removed several years earlier. The site of the operation was where I felt the heat sensation. The scar was hidden by a brassiere, so I had no visual clue. Two weeks later, perhaps made more observant by the first case, I felt a similar heat sensation over an abdominal scar in a different patient.

These two cases led me to use my hands often to feel for heat radiating from the bodies of patients. At first I focused on patients with known pathologies previously identified by other testing methods. After my hands were somewhat "trained" through this experience, I applied this technique to all patients.

I made it a habit to evaluate thermal flow by holding my hands near, but not in contact with, the patient's body. Experience showed that a hand held near the body can make minute discriminations of radiant temperature, whereas its thermosensitivity is muddled when it is placed directly on the skin.

Principles of manual thermal diagnosis

Over the years I have practiced manual thermal diagnosis (MTD) with tens of thousands of patients having a wide variety of diseases or disorders. Gradually, from this experience, I have constructed a thermal "topographic map." Characteristic thermal projections can be correlated with specific disorders and symptoms. MTD makes it possible to locate pathologies quickly and efficiently.

Although primarily a technique for localization of disease, MTD also serves to determine structural abnormalities and other problems. To use it, the practitioner obviously needs to develop manual sensitivity, yet this by itself is not sufficient. One cannot treat a patient effectively without an understanding of the structure and functions of the human body. In other words, MTD cannot be used without solid training in anatomy and physiology.

Through both clinical observations and controlled experiments, I have demonstrated that the hand is sensitive to infrared radiation. This thermosensitivity is combined with acute mechanosensitivity. If, as I suspect, the hand can sense lower–frequency portions of the electromagnetic spectrum (e.g. microwaves and possibly radio waves), the potential precision of MTD is essentially limitless.

During a normal clinical evaluation, even by a well–trained practitioner, the conscious mind of the patient typically influences to a large extent the diagnosis. This is because the patient describes what is important to them and the practitioner obtains information about the symptoms and the nature of the problem filtered through the patient's mind. MTD provides a means for the body itself to express its conflicts and problems directly.

In the human body, there are thousands of factors capable of causing disruption and perturbation. It is of course impossible to examine each one specifically. MTD is a form of general examination "by ambush," where the hand can be thought of as "lying in wait" for messages sent by the body.

All tissues and functions of the body, including the emotions, give rise to characteristic types of thermal flow when they are disrupted. In this book, I will try to describe ways I have learned to sense and understand these thermal flows and their causes.

CHAPTER 2

Heat and Infrared

THIS CHAPTER will cover a few elementary physical concepts relating to temperature. Osteopaths, of course, are more accustomed to working with their hands than with mathematics or physics. To ensure that the text is understandable and useful to the reader, I will define even the simplest and most basic terms.

ENERGY AND HEAT

Energy is the physical factor needed for producing work, and is essential for every physical and biophysical mechanism. Heat, one form of energy, is an end product of numerous metabolic and mechanical transformations that take place in an organism.

Whereas plants obtain energy from the sun, animals obtain energy from food. In animal cells, energy is transformed by oxidation of food materials. This is the most basic type of work done in the human body.

THERMAL FUNCTION IN ORGANISMS

Endothermic or homeothermic ("warm-blooded") animals, i.e. mammals and birds, have evolved physiological mechanisms to maintain internal temperature within a narrow range regardless of external temperatures. Ectotherms (e.g. reptiles, amphibians, insects) have evolved various behavioral means of thermoregulation, but ultimately their internal temperature is dependent upon the external environment and can vary widely. Homeothermy is based on numerous metabolic processes all directed at maintaining a constant body temperature. Heat produced in the body is transmitted to the external environment via the skin when core temperature exceeds external temperature.

The temperature of a given part of the body is the result of metabolic activity in all surrounding tissues. Different regions and organs of the body have slightly different temperatures.

Infrared radiation

Infrared is the term applied to electromagnetic (EM) radiation with a greater wavelength and lower frequency than that of visible red light. The range of wavelength for infrared is defined as 800 to 1000 nanometers (nm) (Illustration 2-1). One nanometer is 10^{-9} m, or one-billionth of a meter. The range for microwaves begins at 1250 nm.

The visible spectrum extends only from 400 nm (violet) to 800 nm (red). Therefore, the human eye is not able to detect infrared.

All bodies give off EM radiation in the form of waves. Some EM waves are capable of transporting thermal energy. Heat energy, as dissipated by or sensed by the human body, is carried by radiation in the infrared range.

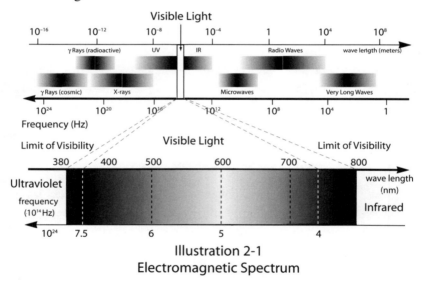

Illustration 2-1
Electromagnetic Spectrum

Definition of period

The period of a defined phenomenon is the duration from beginning to end of the phenomenon. Period is measured in units of time (milliseconds, seconds, minutes, etc.). For example, if the phenomenon being discussed is a heartbeat, and we observe that there are 60 heartbeats per minute, we can say that the period of one heartbeat is one second. EM waves have periods considerably less than one second.

Definition of frequency

The frequency of a repeating phenomenon with defined period is the number of repetitions of the phenomenon per unit time. For the heartbeat example above, we could say that the frequency is 60 repetitions per minute, or one repetition per second. For EM waves, the commonly used unit is Hertz (Hz), defined as number of repetitions per second. Frequency of EM radiation is independent of medium (i.e. it is the same in air as in a vacuum), and is therefore characteristic of a particular type of radiation. Frequency is shown along the bottom of the bands in Illustration 2-1. Notice that infrared radiation has frequencies between roughly 10^{12} to 10^{14} Hz, i.e. there are 10^{12} to 10^{14} waves per second.

Definition of wavelength

The wavelength of an EM wave in a vacuum is the distance it travels during a length of time equal to its period. In Illustration 2-1, wavelength (measured in m or nm) is shown along the top of the bands. Notice that wavelength is inversely proportional to frequency, i.e. the shorter the wavelength, the higher the frequency. As mentioned above, visible light has wavelengths between 400 and 800 nm, while infrared has wavelengths between 800 and 1000 nm.

Transmission of heat

Thermodynamics

When a hot object is placed in cold water, the temperature of the object decreases while the temperature of the water increases until the object and the water are "in equilibrium," i.e. have the same temperature. In general, when two bodies of unequal temperature are in contact, energy is transmitted (i.e. heat flows) from the warmer body toward the colder body. This basic law of thermodynamics is of great interest for our purposes here. When the internal temperature of the human body is greater than that of the surrounding air, as is usually the case, heat is transmitted from the body to the exterior via exposed skin surfaces.

Heat transmission between "body" and skin

Anatomically speaking, the skin is part of the body. In fact, it is the largest and heaviest organ of the body. For our purposes in this book, however, we need to differentiate between the skin and the rest of the body. Although it may be confusing, I will hereafter use the term "body" to refer to all human tissues and organs except the epithelial layer of the skin (epidermis) and its underlying connective tissue layer (dermis). In other words, the word "body" will refer to all living tissues situated deep to the skin, i.e. muscles, blood, bone, digestive organs, lungs, etc.

The heat of the body is transmitted to the skin by conduction, convection, and radiation (also known as radiance).

Conduction

Conduction is the transmission of heat between two solid objects through direct contact, or through a medium without perceptible motion of the medium itself.

Tissue conduction occurs when two tissues of unequal temperature are in contact. Heat is conducted from the warmer to the colder tissue. Normally, heat is conducted from the interior body toward the fasciae near the surface, toward the epidermis, and finally to the exterior.

Convection

In convection, there are currents or movement in a liquid or gas medium, and these currents transfer heat from one region to another. For example, blood is a liquid medium which moves and carries heat.

In general, the difference between conduction and convection involves type of matter (solid versus liquid or air) and molecular currents within the matter (absent versus present).

- Natural convection: Liquid molecules (e.g. in the body) move in response to density differentials created by temperature changes.
- Forced convection: Some force acts on liquid or gas molecules to displace them. Movement of molecules may be turbulent (in many directions) or laminar (mostly in one direction).

- Convection via blood flow: More heat transfer occurs by this route than by direct conduction between tissues. Blood picks up heat as it flows through an active muscle or internal organ. The heat is transmitted to the skin, which loses it to the exterior since temperature of the air is usually lower than that of the skin. Variation in skin temperature is usually felt by the hand as a zone of relative heat, even though thermal recordings may indicate a hypothermic zone.

Radiation

Radiation is an electromagnetic phenomenon sharing some of the properties of light. It is a process of energy propagation involving emission of EM waves or particles. It is characterized by its nature, its energy (expressed in volts), and its flow. Flow (sometimes called flux) means the number of particles striking a unit surface area per unit time.

The skin is an efficient radiator of heat energy. The wavelengths emitted cover a broad spectrum. According to Wien's Law, the frequency at which maximal energy is emitted depends on the temperature of the emitting object. At 37°C (body temperature), radiation from human skin is maximal at a wavelength around 950–1000 nm, i.e. toward the high end of the infrared portion of the EM spectrum (Illustration 2-1). J. D. Hardy (1961) showed that around 30°C maximal skin radiation is at wavelengths between 900 and 1000 nm.

Radiation, as an EM phenomenon, does not rely on the molecules of its medium (e.g. air). It occurs even in a vacuum. It is not greatly affected by the temperature of the medium. For example, your skin can feel the radiant heat from an infrared lamp even if the intervening air is cold.

Although wavelengths of radiation from the skin are strongest in the infrared portion of the spectrum, other wavelengths (from a few hundred nm to several meters) are also given off. Of special interest are frequencies in the range of one to 10 GHz, as we will see later.

An object with a temperature near that of the body, let's say 33°C, also emits radiation primarily in the infrared range. At these wavelengths the skin acts something like a "black body," emitting and absorbing radiation at a coefficient near one. An idealized black body absorbs all the radiation that reaches it.

Skin emissivity

The skin radiates energy toward the objects which surround it, and these objects conversely radiate toward the skin. Many parameters affect these exchanges of radiation: shapes, colors, temperatures, and emissivity of the objects involved.

The emissivity of skin depends on which part of the infrared range we are talking about. For wavelengths around 950 nm, the emissivity of skin is close to that of a black body (i.e. coefficient near one). When skin lacks its normal consistency, or particularly when the surrounding air is humid, the emissivity coefficient is diminished.

As wavelength gets farther from 950 nm, emissivity coefficient of the skin gets farther from one. This is responsible for the colors that we see. In the visible range of EM radiation (between 400 and 800 nm), emissivity and absorption of skin are low (Hardy, 1961). A light-skinned person has lower skin emissivity than a dark-skinned person.

Summary

The skin emits EM radiation. Maximal energy is emitted at wavelengths around 950 nm, in the infrared portion of the EM spectrum.

For our purposes, the skin (epidermis and dermis) may be viewed as an electrical resistor or insulator between the body and the exterior. This insulator slows down heat exchange by convection and conduction, but is a good conductor of infrared radiation.

CHAPTER 3

Body Temperature

Before one can use manual thermal diagnosis, it is necessary to have an understanding of the body temperature. In this chapter I will introduce some of the basic information about the temperatures of different parts of the body and how they vary over time. This will give us a framework upon which to build a thermal picture of the body.

General Body Temperature

Homeothermy and poikilothermy

Birds and mammals, including man, are classified as endotherms (body temperature is based on internal metabolic processes) and homeotherms (core body temperature is relatively constant). In contrast, reptiles, fish, and most invertebrates are classified as ectotherms (body temperature is based on external environment) and poikilotherms (core temperature can vary widely).

In reality, of course, human core (body) temperature (which I shall abbreviate hereafter as TB) can vary somewhat as a function of physical activity, fever, hormonal actions, emotional status, etc. Tissues in the arms and legs, or near the surface of the torso, are often cooler than those deep in the torso (Illustration 3-1). Nevertheless, in comparison to a typical ectotherm (snake, grasshopper), humans can be regarded as maintaining a fairly constant TB.

Body and skin

In human thermal physics the word "core" is often used in opposition to skin. As explained in Chapter 2, I prefer to use the word "body" ("organisme" in French) instead of "core" when referring to temperatures below the skin. Average TB for humans is 37°C. There is certainly

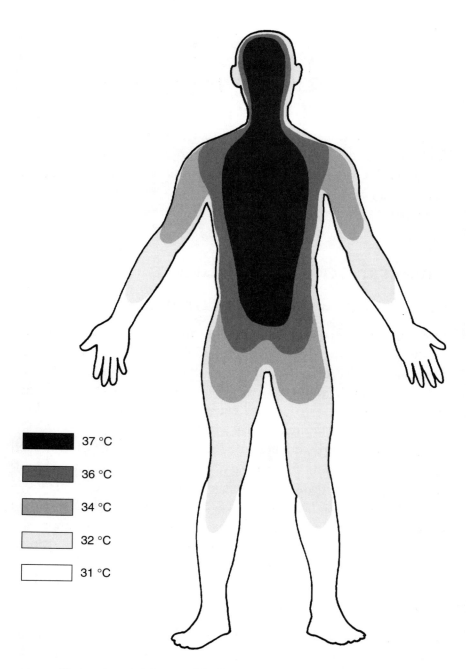

Illustration 3-1: Internal Differences in Body Temperature (Environmental Temperature of ~22°C)

variability, as mentioned above. On a cold day, the temperature of your feet may be 5° less than that inside the abdomen. During digestion of a heavy meal, temperature of blood entering the liver may rise to 40°. Each organ is thermally distinct from its neighbor. An average value for a body at rest with "room temperature" surroundings is 37°C.

Physiological sources of thermal change

A few important factors which can change TB are described here.

Age

TB of a fetus is higher than that of its mother. After birth, temperature quickly decreases. There can be a slight increase during "growth spurts" and usually there is a decrease after adolescence. A slight increase may occur at menopause, and a decrease in old age, especially with reduced activity.

Circadian rhythm

There is a circadian (daily) variation in TB of about 0.5°C. The maximum is usually around 6 PM and the minimum (which corresponds to highest parasympathetic activity) around 3–4 AM. Interestingly, in experiments where humans were placed in conditions of exaggerated isolation (decreased stimulation from light, noise, etc.), the timing and degree of highest daily temperature remained the same.

Menstrual cycle

In the average adult female, TB is ~36.5°C in the postmenstrual (pre-ovulatory) phase. It falls briefly to 36.1° around day 14 of a typical 28-day cycle, in association with the luteinizing hormone "surge" which triggers ovulation. Temperature then climbs rapidly to 37° by day 16 and stays there throughout the postovulatory phase, under the influence of progesterone and estradiol released by the corpus luteum. As the corpus luteum degenerates and hormone levels fall, TB also falls rapidly back to 36.5° in association with the onset of the menstrual phase.

Digestion and metabolic activity

Heat released when food is being digested in the small intestine raises TB by 0.1–0.2°C. Alcohol intake has the same effect. Increased metabolic activity of any sort tends to increase TB, since heat is being released by cells. Heavy exercise (e.g. running) can raise TB as high as 40°C.

Male versus female

Men and women have different TB mainly because of two factors: hormonal differences and a lower basal metabolic rate in women. The latter allows women to more easily achieve internal thermal equilibrium. On the other hand, it also causes women relative difficulty in adapting to large changes in external temperature.

Emotion

Intense emotion usually increases TB. Occasionally, it has the opposite effect. The reasons for this are unclear.

Regional differences in temperature

The body exchanges heat with the outside environment via the skin. Different regions of the body, or the skin, have different temperatures. The temperature of a given region or organ depends on a constantly changing balance between heat production and heat loss. In general, the body maintains its temperature within a narrower range than the skin. When a pathology exists, the skin reflects the thermal disequilibrium of the body.

Average heat production varies from organ to organ. We can organize the organs into groups having similar thermal properties (see Chapter 5).

Heat transfer by blood

The bloodstream is primarily responsible for heat transfer within the body. Heat loss from an organ is a function of the quantity of blood passing through it, and local tonus of the blood vessels. Thermal equilibrium of an organ depends largely on the temperature of entering blood.

Arteries and veins

Except in the extremities, venous blood is almost always warmer than arterial blood. This appears to be attributable to metabolites released into venous blood, and the fact that heat itself is a waste product of oxidation in cells. In the thorax, the increase in venous temperature is progressive, moving upward along the inferior vena cava to the right atrium. Although the temperature of arterial blood may be higher than that of surrounding tissues, in the trunk and head blood is progressively cooled in the arteries and warmed in the veins—contrary to what most people would guess (Houdas and Guieu, 1977; Houdas and Ring, 1982).

Extremities

It is not uncommon for temperatures in the extremities (particularly the hands or feet) to be 10°C less than in the thorax. In the arms and legs, arteries are often in very close proximity to their corresponding veins. As a result, heat from the arterial blood (which is flowing away from the trunk) is progressively transferred, by conduction, to nearby venous blood (which is flowing toward the trunk) (Illustration 3-2). This mechanism, known as countercurrent heat exchange, is found in many vertebrates and is a good way to avoid losing body heat to the external environment. By the time it reaches the fingers and toes, arterial blood may have cooled considerably, resulting in lower temperature of surrounding tissues and skin. Degree of conduction between adjacent tissues depends on the temperature gradient between them, and their conductibility (a characteristic physical property).

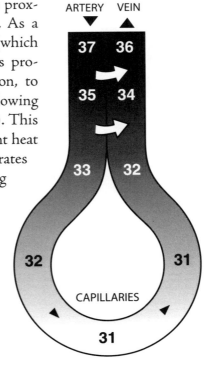

Illustration 3-2: Temperature of the Extremities.

Scrotum

Normal function of the testes requires a local temperature that is lower than TB. If the testes become too warm, sperm production declines. The scrotum holds the testes away from the rest of the abdomen and allows them to stay cooler. But this is not the only cooling mechanism. The testicular artery is close to the testicular vein, allowing significant countercurrent heat exchange. The skin surface of the scrotum can be contracted or distended, under control of the nervous system. The surface area decreases in response to cold and increases in response to heat; degree of heat exchange with the exterior is correspondingly decreased or increased. Through these mechanisms, the temperature inside the testes is maintained at not more than 34.5°C, while that at the surface of the scrotum is usually 32–33°C.

Abdominal organs

Temperature of these organs is related to their metabolic activity. Following ingestion of alcohol or fatty foods, the liver becomes metabolically very active and its temperature may rise to 40°C. At rest, its temperature is about the same as that of the stomach or kidneys.

The rectum, at a depth of 8cm, has a relatively high temperature. This may be due to the numerous veins that surround the rectum and low blood flow in the pelvis.

The temperature of the stomach is naturally variable depending on what has been recently ingested. If you eat ice cream, or drink hot coffee, the stomach may go down to 22°C or up to 40°C.

Brain

The brain, along with the heart, is the most crucial organ. The circulatory system is designed to ensure a steady supply of blood to the brain, and thereby protect it against major decreases in temperature or oxygen supply, even at the expense of the rest of the body. Recently, the temperature of the brain has been deduced from measurements of the temperature of the inner ear.

The hypothalamus, which forms the floor and part of the lateral walls of the third ventricle in the brain, is the control center for TB. Certain cells in the hypothalamus function as thermostats, responding to the temperature of incoming blood. If blood temperature is too high or too low, the hypothalamus can produce appropriate corrections in the body via the autonomic nervous system. For example, it can promote heat loss through vasodilation (relaxation of smooth muscle) of cutaneous blood vessels, leading to heat loss through the skin, or through sweating. It can promote heat retention through vasoconstriction or shivering.

It has been noted that the temperature of the inner ear recovers relatively quicker than that of other parts of the body after a sudden fall in temperature. Perhaps the proximity of the hypothalamus to this area offers an explanation.

Diagnostic consideration

Different regions of the body and skin have different temperatures. However, certain skin regions are less variable than others. In MTD, we utilize both variable and constant regions in localizing pathologies, as will be shown in subsequent chapters.

CHAPTER 4

Skin Temperature

IN MTD, skin temperature (abbreviated hereafter as T_S) is our primary tool for localizing pathological zones. Heat transfer between the body and the exterior occurs via the skin. Certain regions of the body typically have higher rates of heat transfer than others. In MTD, we are less concerned with absolute T_S than with relative T_S, especially comparing one side against the other.

Variations in T_S

When ambient temperature (hereafter T_A) is lower than T_B, much of the heat produced by the body is lost to the exterior via the skin. The respiratory system and sweating play lesser roles in heat loss.

In a state of thermal stability, heat transfer from the skin to the exterior is the same as that from the body to the skin, and T_S reflects what is happening inside the body. T_S in a given location depends on the conductibility of subcutaneous tissue. Some lesions have a higher metabolic level and higher conductibility than surrounding normal tissues. According to Houdas and Ring (1982), "The skin which covers these zones has a more elevated temperature than the adjoining skin." These authors state that this phenomenon is detectable only when the lesion is near the skin. However, my clinical and experimental experience suggests otherwise. With a lesion of the kidney, an organ situated deeply in the retroperitoneal region, T_S at the abdominal surface projection is elevated. This can be explained by heat radiation.

Heat transfer through the skin

T_S is generally between 32 and 33°C. When T_A is lower than T_S, heat is transferred from the skin to the exterior. How does heat from the body reach the skin in the first place? The three mechanisms are the ones already defined in Chapter 2: conduction, convection, and radiation.

Conduction

Warming of the skin may occur via conduction. Heat is produced by muscles and all metabolically active organs and can be transferred to contiguous tissues. By its nature, warming by conduction is most notable for tissues in direct contact with the heat–producing area. Consider an inflammation or ulcer in the duodenum. The affected area becomes warmer. The greater omentum, rectus abdominis muscle, and overlying skin also become warmer.

Warming of the skin by conduction is a function of the conductibility of subcutaneous tissue. Conductibility of pathological zones is often elevated, which helps explain why overlying Ts is also relatively high.

Convection and the bloodstream

Much of the transfer of heat from body to skin is via the bloodstream. TS at a particular region depends in part on the amount of blood flow reaching that region.

I mentioned in Chapter 3 that, within the body, arterial blood tends to cool surrounding tissues and venous blood tends to warm them. However, at the skin level venous blood is usually cooler than arterial blood. Heat from arterial blood, not venous blood, is transferred to the skin and thence to the exterior.

The amount of heat reaching the skin depends on volume of blood flow as well as temperature of the blood. Flow volume is regulated by constriction or dilation of vessels, under control of the autonomic nervous system. Every change in blood flow results in a change in Ts. This applies to cutaneous regions above or connected to pathogenic zones such as tumors or dysfunctional sphincters.

By modifying cutaneous vasomotor tone, the nervous system can modify Ts. This explains the rapidity with which Ts can change.

Blood vessels, glomera, and vasodilation

Blood vessels are found only in the dermis, not the epidermis. Arteries terminate in arterioles and metarterioles, both of which give rise to capillaries. Sometimes capillaries form complex branching networks, which increase surface area available for diffusion of materials or heat transfer. After passing through the capillaries, blood is collected by venules and then veins.

A glomus (plural glomera) is a tiny, well-innervated ball-like structure composed of arterioles which connect directly with venules. Glomera are found almost everywhere, but are most numerous in the extremities. Vessel diameter in glomera is under sympathetic nervous control and can vary from 0 to ~70μm, causing blood to either pass through capillaries or be "short-circuited" through the glomera.

Glomera are thought to be the site of vasodilation leading to localized hyperthermia. In general, vasodilation occurs in regions having a high density of glomera. There are ~500 glomera per cm^2 beneath the fingernails, $115/cm^2$ at the thenar eminence, and $95/cm^2$ at the hypothenar eminence.

Vasodilation has important local and systemic effects:
- increased blood flow at the skin
- increased T_S
- increased temperature gradient between skin and exterior
- increased loss of heat from the skin and body.

Vasoconstriction results in decrease of each of the above parameters.

Vasomotor control

Vasodilation is controlled by the sympathetic nervous system. It results from decreased tone (contraction) of smooth muscle fibers in the walls of glomera or other vessels. Widespread vasodilation occurs after vigorous exercise or in a hot climate. If a small region of skin is heated, vasodilation does not appear only at that region. Vasomotor control is based on integrated information or input from the skin, body, and hypothalamus.

Sweat

Sweat (sudoriferous) glands have their secretory portion located in the dermis or subcutaneous layer. The excretory duct opens into a hair follicle or a pore at the surface of the epidermis. Sweat (perspiration), the liquid released by these glands, is a mixture of water, salts, urea, amino acids, lactic acid, and other substances. Evaporation of sweat helps cool the skin.

I have tried to determine whether a relationship exists between the zones of perspiration and pathogenic zones. Such a relationship may exist, but it is certainly less obvious than that of cutaneous hyperthermic zones.

Radiation

Skin emissivity varies with wavelength. As mentioned in Chapter 2, at ~950 nm (infrared range), skin emissivity is like that of a black body, i.e. it absorbs essentially all radiation. The wavelengths of radiation striking or emitted by the skin range from a few hundred nm to several meters. I believe that receptors in the hand are sensitive to a wide range of EM wavelengths. There is substantial proof for palpation of infrared radiation. Further research is needed on other parts of the EM spectrum.

Sensitivity to microwaves

Radiation from the skin includes wavelengths shorter than infrared (e.g. visible light) and longer than infrared (e.g. microwaves). The intensity of microwaves from human skin is about 108 times weaker than that of infrared radiation. Human tissue is partially transparent to microwaves. It is possible in theory to detect microwave emissions from skin or subcutaneous tissues and measure their intensity (Houdas and Ring, 1982). Instruments for this purpose have been constructed utilizing antennae that are usually put in contact with the skin, to eliminate reflections between the skin and surrounding air. Sometimes the antennae are clear of the skin. Such instruments have been able to detect changes in intensity corresponding to variations in emitted temperature on the order of 0.1°C. This variation is similar to that which the hand can detect by palpating infrared radiation from skin.

When palpating infrared from skin, the hand feels an impression of (1) warmth, and (2) a difference in intensity (or "pressure") of radiation. The reason for this is unclear at present. Is it due to differential activation of thermal receptors in the hand, the perception of other EM waves, a combination of these factors, or some other factor?

Regional variation in T_S

The skin and subcutaneous layer may be regarded as a "thermal resistance" barrier between the body and exterior. About 10 percent of cardiac output reaches the skin. Skin can act to "dampen" thermal variations by reducing thermal flow, except over underlying zones of conflict.

Heat production by the skin itself is relatively minor, often considered as zero. When T_A is lower than T_S, T_S generally reflects T_B. As mentioned above, every change of cutaneous blood flow results in a variation of T_S, and the nervous system regulates T_S via vasomotor tone.

Physicians and physiologists usually look at overall variations in T_S, not local variation between one region and another. However, the local variations reflect internal conditions, and allow us to localize pathological zones.

"Average" T_S

This has been calculated repeatedly by me and many other authors. Average T_S lies between 32 and 35°C, except at the extremities. For skin surfaces that are large and relatively flat (e.g. abdomen, thorax), variations in T_S are slight. On the other hand, T_S at an extremity (e.g. cold feet) may be 10°C less than at a warm region such as the armpit.

Natural hypothermic regions

Extremities

When T_A is considerably lower than T_B, values of T_S for the extremities (particularly the feet) are typically lower than for other regions.

Countercurrent heat exchange was explained in Chapter 3. This phenomenon can also lead to lower T_S at the extremities, including the scrotum.

Other

Other relatively hypothermic regions include the breasts, buttocks, cellulite bundles, and stretch marks. Scars are usually hypothermic, except when they create abnormal mechanical tensions. When the intestines or stomach contain excessive gas, their surface projections can be hypothermic.

Female/male difference

At room temperature, women have lower T_S than men. Apparent causative factors are higher cutaneous vasomotor tone, lower metabolic rate, and better "thermal resistance" (insulation) by the subcutaneous layer in women.

NATURAL HYPERTHERMIC REGIONS

These include natural skin folds (e.g., elbows, knees, axillae, inferior aspect of breasts in contact with thorax), cutaneous folds in obese subjects, the superomedial thighs, and the suboccipital region.

CIRCADIAN PATTERN

T_S exhibits circadian thermal variation patterns similar to and slightly preceding those of T_B. This may be explained by the facts that the body usually reacts to external temperature stimuli via the skin, and most thermoreceptors are in the skin.

REMOTE MEASUREMENT OF T_S

In order to have objective confirmation of T_S variations perceived by hand, it was necessary to have a mechanical instrument capable of measuring T_S without contacting the skin. I am very grateful to the engineers Daniel Boutron, François Collomb, and Bernard Million, who worked with me on this long and difficult project. The instrument which they perfected has been indispensable for gathering data and establishing MTD on an objective basis.

Thermal zones in humans

Data I have collected on tens of thousands of subjects reveal that the human skin surface can be divided into fairly distinct thermal zones or compartments, as shown in Illustration 4-1. Within each of these zones, assuming no pathology exists, Ts measured remotely by hand or instrument does not vary significantly from one point to another.

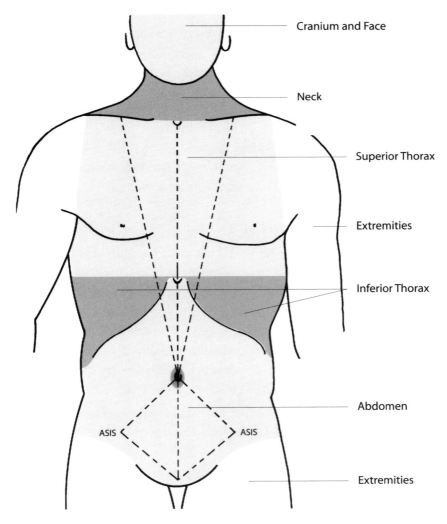

Illustration 4-1: Cutaneous Thermal Zones

The concept of these thermal zones guides our comparative studies. It serves no purpose to compare Ts in the thorax to that of the abdomen, since these are different zones and naturally have different values. On the other hand, *within* the thorax (or any other zone), one point may be meaningfully compared to another.

Anterior thermal zones, shown in the illustration, are:
- cranium and face
- neck
- upper thorax (bordered inferiorly by ribs 5 and 6 on the right and left respectively)
- lower thorax (bordered inferiorly by the bottom rib)
- abdomen
- arms and legs.

Experience has shown that in MTD the hand may pass without difficulty from one zone to another. As in so many other functions, the brain adapts very quickly, and the sensing hand can thus adapt to differences in "background" Ts in a fraction of a second.

Adaptation to change in T_A

In response to sudden changes in T_A, there is typically a transitional period during which Ts falls or rises, eventually reaching a new equilibrium value. After equilibrium is reached, the usual differences among thermal zones persist. The time needed to adapt (reach new equilibrium Ts value) is generally around five minutes, but may be much longer for hypothermic regions such as the feet.

Unusually high or low T_A obviously interferes with MTD. Ts is most "expressive" (suitable for MTD) when T_A is around 22–23°C.

Significance of variations in Ts

As mentioned above, heat production by the skin is insignificant compared to that of muscles and other metabolically active organs. When variations in Ts are detected, they are due to heat production not by the skin, but rather by tissues or organs beneath the skin. Once you have learned to compensate for the normal variations between different thermal zones, you will be able to recognize the variations in Ts which reflect internal dysfunctions or pathologies.

For example, when there is inflammation of the antrum or pylorus, resulting heat is transmitted by conduction to neighboring tissues such as the jejunum and ileum, greater omentum, right rectus abdominis and its aponeurosis, dermis, and epidermis. Cutaneous vasodilation occurs and Ts at the surface projection of the inflamed area increases. The degree of Ts increase reflects the degree of underlying inflammation.

What type of radiation?

It seems likely that heat transfer as described above involves mostly EM radiation in the infrared range. As mentioned previously, skin is like a black body for infrared, i.e. it absorbs nearly all infrared radiation.

On the other hand, it is possible to perform MTD through clothing (though with greater difficulty than over bare skin). This is interesting because clothing blocks most infrared. I believe that other wavelengths above or below the infrared range are passing through, and our hands are able to detect them (though perhaps with less sensitivity than infrared). Further research is needed to test the validity of this idea.

CHAPTER 5

Thermal Control and Regulation

Cells that respond to changes in temperature, and send this information to the central nervous system (CNS), are called "thermoreceptors." The amount of information that reaches the CNS depends on the number of thermoreceptors activated, intensity of the stimulus, and duration of the stimulus. Human skin contains specific thermoreceptors for heat and cold. Sensitivity to heat is a property of almost all living cells. This property is most important for cells which have a low response threshold.

Thermal control is achieved through feedback loops which involve thermoreceptors, heat-regulating centers in the brain, and motor (effector) neurons.

T_B is relatively but not absolutely constant. It varies slightly in response to physical activity, T_A, hormone levels, circadian cycles, and other factors discussed in Chapter 4. There are also variations from one region to another.

"Overall" T_B is not affected by increased or decreased temperature of a single organ, e.g. the cecum. Control of T_B is a systemic (global) phenomenon. There are always local relative excesses of heat.

Thermoreceptors

Thermoreceptors are located not only in the skin but also internally. Thermoreceptors in the viscera are located within the organs themselves. I believe that mechanoreceptors in the fasciae can also serve as thermoreceptors.

Peripheral thermoreceptors

Specialized Ruffini's corpuscles (sensitive to heat) and Krause's corpuscles (sensitive to cold) are located in the dermis. Both can produce sensations of pain if overstimulated. Free nerve endings located just below the epidermis (or between cells of the basal layer) also show thermal sensitivity, particularly to cold.

Signals from dermal thermoreceptors are relayed to spinal ganglia and from there to the lateral part of the posterior gray horn of the spinal cord. These fibers end on neurons of the substantia gelatinosa or the ventrolateral column.

Receptors in the skin are functionally segregated. Receptors for pain and touch are most superficial. Those for temperature are intermediate. Those for pressure are deepest.

Afferent fibers which relay signals from these various receptors may be bundled together. At the level of the posterior horn of the spinal cord, their territory is more clearly differentiated.

The proximity of thermoreceptors and mechanoreceptors in the dermis is interesting. I suspect that mechanical stimuli can lead to heat messages.

Activity of peripheral thermoreceptors

Thermoreceptors in the skin are "tuned" to respond to certain temperature ranges. The signals they send to the CNS lead to our conscious perception of T_A. Physiological responses to increases or decreases in T_A are mediated by the CNS.

We can consider two types of response by peripheral thermoreceptors.
- Static: A thermoreceptor in a stable state generates a certain number of impulses per second. There is a characteristic, nonlinear relationship between the receptor's temperature and its firing frequency. Heat receptors increase their firing frequency as the skin is heated from 25 to 40°C. Their frequency falls at temperatures above 45°C (burning).

  In contrast, cold receptors increase their firing frequency as the skin is cooled from 38 to 30°C. Frequency then falls at lower temperatures.
- Dynamic: When T_A changes rapidly, firing frequency of thermoreceptors does not immediately reach its new level. Rate of change in the frequency can vary depending on the magnitude

and rapidity of change in T$_A$. There is an important difference between heat and cold receptors. As T$_A$ increases, frequency of heat receptors may temporarily "overshoot" its final, relatively stable, level. Cold receptors exhibit a more steady increase in frequency as T$_A$ falls.

Density and properties of peripheral thermoreceptors

Density depends on location. It is higher in the face (including ears and tongue) and scrotum. In terms of overall numbers, the skin contains 10–15 times as many cold receptors as heat receptors.

"Proportional" receptors specifically respond to temperature magnitude. "Differential" receptors are sensitive to the acceleration or rate of temperature change. There are also "mixed" receptors, which combine these two properties. Receptor sensitivity is greatest, and physiological adaptation most efficient, for T$_A$ in the range of 20 to 40°C.

Afferent fibers from heat receptors belong to group C. Cold signals may be carried by group C fibers and by the faster group A fibers.

CENTRAL THERMORECEPTORS

Heating or cooling of the CNS induces systemic (global) temperature control responses (Thauer 1970; Simon 1974). There are primary thermoreceptors in the spinal cord and the hypothalamus (see Chapter 3). There are also numerous centers in the spinal cord, thalamus, hypothalamus, and cortex which respond to information from cutaneous thermoreceptors.

Afferent signals may undergo transformation (inhibition, summation, or exaggeration) during the passage through the spinal cord to the brain. Such transformation may explain the hypersensitivity to T$_A$ changes observed in some patients.

Lateral spinothalamic tract

Afferent fibers from receptors of pain, temperature, pressure, and touch cross into the opposite side of the spinal cord. The lateral spinothalamic tract is an ascending tract which carries sensations of heat and pain of proprioceptive and exteroceptive origin. It passes to the thalamus via the brain stem. As its fibers also carry pain messages from the viscera, such pain is sometimes referred to the area of skin served by the same spinal segment (Head's zones). These zones can become hypersensitive and hyperreactive to touch, pain, or heat.

Thermal and pain messages carried by the lateral spinothalamic tract terminate in the posterior ventral nuclei of the thalamus. So do many other sensory and epicritic pathways. Thus, there is opportunity for "mixing up" of stimuli both at their origin (the peripheral receptors) and at their terminus (the thalamic nuclei). A mechanical stimulus may give a thermal sensation, and vice versa.

Hypothalamus

Only about 25 percent of neurons in the hypothalamus which exhibit sensitivity to heat are considered primary thermoreceptors. These are situated mainly in the preoptic region and generate signals in response to changes in their own temperature. Some of them seem to modify their level of sensitivity as the temperature around them changes. Some hypothalamic neurons produce a thermal response when they receive electrical stimuli which are not related to heat.

In contrast to the skin, the hypothalamus contains far fewer cold receptors than heat receptors.

Mesencephalon (midbrain)

This part of the brain, located between the thalamus and pons, consists of the corpora quadrigemina and cerebral peduncles. It contains many neurons which exhibit high thermal sensitivity. It has been estimated that 79 percent of these are primary heat receptors, 8 percent are primary cold receptors, and 13 percent are interneurons.

Mechanoreceptors

Specialists such as Hardy (1961) and Houdas (1982) have considered the question of how the CNS differentiates afferent impulses of mechanical origin from those of thermal origin. Studies have suggested that when any afferent fiber transmits a mechanical stimulus from a tendon, muscle, fascia, etc., the signal can be transformed into thermal information in the medulla. The mechanism for this is unknown.

Cutaneous mechanoreceptors

Tactile corpuscles (Meissner's corpuscles)

These are most numerous in the palms, pads of the fingers, and soles of the feet. They detect five tactile sensations. They are more receptive to the speed of variation in stimulus intensity than to the intensity itself.

These nerve endings are surrounded by a fine capsule of collagenous fibers. These fibers are continuous with the tonofibrils of the epidermis and are therefore able to easily pick up mechanical deformations of the epidermis.

Tactile menisci (Merkel's cells)

Each of these cup-shaped nerve endings is in contact with a single, modified epithelial cell. They are found in the deep epidermis, hair follicles, and the hard palate. These slow-adapting mechanoreceptors are sensitive to constant pressure.

Lamellar corpuscles (Vater-Pacini corpuscles)

These are structurally the largest (up to 4mm in length) and most complex nerve endings, consisting of many concentric lamellae (layers) of connective tissue. They are found in the deeper layers of the dermis, periosteum, tendons, and serous membranes. They respond to vibrations as well as deep pressure.

Other receptors

There are many other nerve endings which are surrounded by some sort of connective tissue capsule. Bulboid corpuscles (Krause's corpuscles) are found in the skin (where they are sensitive to cold), mucous membranes, conjunctiva, and heart. Golgi-Mazzoni corpuscles are tactile corpuscles found in the subcutaneous tissues of the fingers or the surface of tendons. They resemble lamellar corpuscles but with fewer lamellae and more extensively branched nerve fibers. Ruffini's corpuscles, found in the skin and adipose tissue, are sensitive to pressure and heat.

Sensory nerve endings are found not only in the skin, but also in mucous membranes, articular capsules, and fasciae of internal organs, including the viscera. In all these locations, they sense and provide afferent messages to the CNS on pressure, pain, and temperature.

Much research remains to be done in this area. In some experimental animals, cooling or warming the abdomen leads to activation of global heat regulatory mechanisms. Thermosensitive zones may be found throughout the body. Specialized heat-sensitive cells may be found in major vessels, organs, and muscle fibers.

I view heat as a "thermal flow" in which molecules move about to create a characteristic vibratory field. I believe that skin is sensitive to these molecular movements, and that such information relayed by mechanoreceptors is transformed in the spinal cord into "heat messages." In MTD, heat is often perceived as having qualities of intensity and pressure.

Cutaneous thermoregulation

In a resting human, more than 50 percent of generated heat is due to the internal organs and only around 20 percent to the muscles and skin. With intense physical activity, this situation changes dramatically—the proportion of heat generated by the muscles may exceed 90 percent! As mentioned in Chapter 4, the skin plays a major role in dissipating excess heat through vasodilation and sweating.

Vasodilation

The dermis contains blood vessels; the epidermis does not. The vessels in the dermis form a vascular bed approximately 2mm beneath the epidermis. Diameter of the arterioles is controlled by the sympathetic nervous system. Post-ganglionic efferent fibers of this system affect vasoconstrictive and vasodilative receptors, which are located mostly in the skin and kidneys.

In addition, vascular diameter is affected by catecholamines secreted by the adrenal glands. Epinephrine is vasodilative at low concentrations and vasoconstrictive at higher concentrations. Norepinephrine has a constrictive effect.

Vasodilation consists primarily of diminution or suppression of vasoconstrictive tonus imposed by sympathetic stimuli or catecholamines on the circular smooth muscles in the walls of blood vessels.

The mechanism by which vasodilation results in loss of heat was explained in Chapters 3 and 4.

Sweat glands

There are two types of sweat glands. The apocrine type are simple, branched tubular glands restricted to the axillae, pubic hair, and areolae of the breasts. They become active at puberty and produce a relatively viscous secretion which is released into hair follicles. Their thermoregulatory function is minor.

Eccrine sweat glands are simple, coiled tubular glands widespread over most of the skin. They are active throughout life and produce a relatively watery secretion which is released into a pore at the surface of the epidermis. They play a major role in thermoregulation. You have roughly three or four million eccrine sweat glands. Their density is particularly high on the forehead, inner thighs, soles, and palms (up to 3,000 per square inch).

Innervation of sweat glands

There are three types of nerve fibers. A fibers are myelinated, have large diameters, and conduct impulses quickly. B fibers are also myelinated, with intermediate diameter and conduction speed. C fibers are unmyelinated (i.e. incapable of saltatory conduction), with the smallest diameters and slowest speeds. Sweat glands are innervated by type C postganglionic fibers from the sympathetic nervous system. The fibers which activate sweat glands release acetylcholine as a neurotransmitter, in contrast to most sympathetic postganglionic fibers, which release norepinephrine.

Sweat glands in thermoregulation and MTD

Sweat from eccrine glands evaporates on the skin surface and thereby reduces T_S.

I have often looked for correlations between localized sweating and underlying pathological zones. Two problems are that sweat glands are distributed unevenly, and it is difficult to quantify the evaporation of sweat. Yet it is evident that skin is more likely to be moist over certain pathologies, e.g. a sprain, a fracture, or the liver when hepatitis is present.

CHAPTER 6

Manual Thermal Diagnosis

THE PRECEDING chapters have presented background information necessary for understanding and practicing manual thermal diagnosis (MTD). I now turn to the true subject of this book, MTD itself. In MTD, we use our hands to perceive thermal variations in the patient's body or skin, and evaluate the pathological significance of these variations.

General considerations

MTD is performed without contacting the skin. For a long time I attempted to apply MTD with cutaneous contact, but had little success. When the hand is in direct contact with the skin, many factors can interfere with accurate sensing of thermal projections from the skin and body. The skin may be moist, surface contours may make placement of the hand problematic, body hair may disrupt perception, the hand may warm the skin by conduction, etc.

For these reasons, I chose to always perform MTD off the body. Subsequent experience (including some research described later in this chapter) confirmed that this is the best technique.

LETTING THE BODY "TALK" WITH MTD

In general, when a patient consults a health practitioner, the diagnosis is delimited by the ideas of the patient and the practitioner, i.e., both the practitioner's questions and the patient's responses are limited by his or her understanding, prior experiences, and convictions.

MTD offers a considerable advantage:
- MTD allows the body to directly express its problems.
- The patient is interviewed after MTD in order to compare his or her subjective symptoms with the diagnosis.

A thermal variation shows the location of a problem. Thus, the body itself indicates its zones of conflict. The practitioner, after MTD, "fine tunes" the diagnosis by questioning the patient and palpating the heat-projecting zones, which leads to a more detailed interpretation of the thermal projection.

This further refinement, which depends on detailed knowledge and understanding of human anatomy, normal physiology, and pathophysiology, is crucial. For example, just to know that there is some problem in the upper right quadrant of the abdomen is not sufficient. A parenchymal liver problem and a gallbladder problem require very different treatments.

Obviously, it is necessary to perform the standard physical exam and history for a complete picture of the patient and his/her problems.

LOCATION OF PROBLEM

Thermal flow perceived by the hand allows us to localize a zone of conflict. Analysis of the thermal flow provides additional information. It is always the practitioner's medical knowledge which makes it possible to establish a useful diagnosis.

I have thought about using the phrase "manual thermal location" instead of MTD to emphasize that there are two aspects of the process: thermal detection and thermal diagnosis.

PERCEPTION OF THERMAL "INTENSITY"

There are many "shadow zones" in thermal sensing of the skin and body. These are areas where one senses an intensity along with a change in temperature. They are often found at angles or curves where more than one surface can be felt at once. Perhaps in this situation peripheral thermo- and mechanoreceptors have their impulses combined at the level of the spinal cord and thermoreceptive centers of the brain.

The hand does not merely sense heat, but also the quality of heat.

Other MTD practitioners with whom I have spoken share my opinion: beyond the sensation of heat, the hand receives a sensation of intensity. It is as if more cutaneous receptors of the hand are stimulated as the thermal flow becomes stronger, just as more muscle fibers are recruited as contraction of a muscle becomes stronger. The impression of thermal intensity, besides temperature per se, provides important complementary information.

Is the sensation of intensity related to combinations of different EM wavelengths which activate thermoreceptors and mechanoreceptors at the same time? We don't know yet.

Experimental research

I know from experience how easy it is for practitioners to get carried away with little "discoveries" they think they have made. Often, the force of belief can overwhelm one's objectivity. For this reason, my colleagues and I have performed many experiments to assess MTD using objective instruments and techniques.

Experiments with thermal detectors

Various laboratories in France and the United States have made infrared cameras or cutaneous thermal contacts available to us. There are inherent difficulties in using these devices. Infrared cameras are overly sensitive to heat emitted by large branches of circulatory vessels, which complicates localization of heat projecting zones. Cutaneous thermal contacts are overly sensitive to variations in humidity, hairiness, and skin texture or contours.

The Ortomédic Society of Grenoble, France developed a thermal detector to be used without cutaneous contact, and generously made it available to us. This device is capable of detecting thermal gradients of weak amplitude (<10 milliwatts per cm) and variations in Ts on the order of 0.1°C.

We first searched manually for patients' hyperthermic zones, then applied the remote thermal detector. Every time there was thermal variation, the hand felt it, but the detector revealed a surprising phenomenon. The hand feels every thermal variation as a hot zone, even hypothermic areas! This finding was difficult to believe. We performed thousands of tests before accepting this paradoxical conclusion.

In a way, this simplifies the practice of MTD. Since the hand senses all thermal variation as heat, we simply search for excess heat, with the understanding that even hypothermic zones will be perceived as hyperthermic. In fact, at least 70 percent of perceptible thermal variations are hyperthermic.

Experiments with medical instruments

I have used MTD since 1973. During all these years, I have made efforts to confirm and document objectively what my hands sensed. I have used the technologies of ultrasound, fluoroscopy, radiography, CT scan, and Doppler effect to compare with my manual diagnoses.

I can say that in general the hands sense the location of a problem; it is with medical interpretation of the problem that disagreements may arise. Consider, for example, a small, circular thermal projection slightly above and to the right of the navel. Does it represent a small duodenal ulcer, or a stone in the renal pelvis or upper ureter? The existence of the thermal zone is incontestable, but it requires extensive clinical skill and knowledge of the patient to interpret it correctly.

Meaning of thermal variations

Thermal variations are found over what I call "zones of conflict." Significance and interpretation of the thermal zones depends on their configuration and intensity.

For readers whose osteopathic training is different from mine, I would like to clarify some of my basic concepts.

Structural versus functional problems

I have been surprised to observe frequent misunderstandings of these terms in the clinical environment.

- Structural problems: These result from some disorder or crisis of tissue structure. The disorder can be documented objectively by conventional medical techniques. Examples are tumors and ulcers.

- Functional problems: These result from abnormal functioning of a tissue or organ. There is no tissue disorder that can be objectively documented by conventional medical techniques.

A "normal" liver ultrasound does not prove that this organ is functioning in an optimal, healthy manner. A "normal" radiograph of the vertebral column does not prove that it is functioning optimally, or that there is no back pain. Very often migraine headaches have no known organic basis, but are nonetheless real and extremely debilitating.

Unlike most medical techniques, MTD allows us to detect and evaluate the functional problems which lead to almost 85 percent of medical office consultations.

The clinical dilemma

Before becoming structural, a problem typically passes through a functional stage. Only after tens of millions of cells are involved can the problem be documented objectively. Using MTD, I have frequently located and identified pathologies that were first documented by conventional procedures months or even years later. I was often far ahead of even the symptoms.

This can pose a significant ethical dilemma, illustrated by the following example (I have had many similar situations). A female patient consulted for back pain with radiation into the left rib cage area. There were only minimal vertebral restrictions. Using MTD, I detected a very strong thermal projection from the left breast. Attempting to be prudent and cautious, I asked whether the patient had recently consulted her regular physician. She replied, "There can't be anything wrong with me, absolutely nothing. I just had a mammogram three weeks ago."

One year later she had a malignant tumor removed from the left breast.

Should I have insisted on vigorous follow-up at my initial exam in the absence of major warning signs other than MTD? Would this have created cancerphobia and major psychological trauma for her and her family?

Shapes of thermal projections

Thermal projections may be punctiform, small and circular, linear, large and circular, or broad bands. They may have precise or indistinct boundaries.

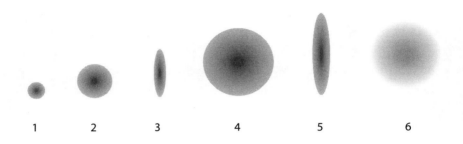

Illustration 6-1: Thermal Configurations

Punctiform and small circular zones: Thermal projections of these types (Illustration 6-1, nos. 1 and 2) may represent precise structural problems such as a calculus or tumor. They may also signify problems of sphincters or sphincter-like structures (e.g. hiatal and pyloric inflammation).

Linear zones: These signify a problem in a small tube (e.g. artery, vein, lymph vessel, bile duct, ureter). The thermal projection is narrow and intense (no. 3).

Large circular zones with precise boundaries: These indicate a problem in an entire organ or a large portion of it (e.g. hepatitis, irritation of gastric mucosa). The thermal projection is wide and intense (no. 4).

Bands: These signify a problem in a large tube-shaped organ (e.g. esophagus, intestine) (no. 5).

Large circular zones without precise boundaries: These indicate a functional (not structural) visceral problem, possibly with an emotion-

al or psychological component (no. 6). For example, when the liver has a structural problem (e.g. hepatitis), the thermal projection is large, but with very well-defined, precise boundaries. A projection over the liver without precise boundaries may reflect either:
- a functional problem. Perhaps there is difficulty (associated with pain) in digesting certain foods. The patient is stressed by having to pay close attention to her diet.
- an emotional thermal zone (see below).

Emotional thermal zones

These projections are often large, sometimes intense, but the boundaries are characteristically vague, changeable, and hard to pinpoint. Emotional zones may appear for various reasons.

STRESS

Stress may be psychological, physical, or behavioral in origin. Emotional reactions to stress may be:
- acute. This includes autonomic reactions such as dyspnea, precordial pain, syncope or feeling of faintness, headache accompanied by vertigo, spastic colon, and vomiting.
- delayed. The reaction is negligible or absent at the time of stress but manifests itself later.
- chronic. The reaction lasts a long time. Examples are recurrent anxiety attacks and vague (but intense) feelings of uneasiness with associated autonomic and behavioral disturbances. Often these reactions are far "out of proportion" to the original stress.

PSYCHOSOMATIC PROBLEMS

Visceral problems of psychosomatic origin are well documented. They range from innocuous headaches to life-threatening hemorrhagic colitis. Other examples are back pain, gastritis, ulcer, asthma, dermatitis, psoriasis, urticaria, hypertension, coronary spasm, and irritable bowel syndrome.

Correlations between organs and emotions

I have seen hundreds of patients who presented with visceral pathologies, and looked for correlations with psychological, behavioral, or emotional phenomena. In some cases I have found evidence for such correlation, as will be mentioned in subsequent chapters.

I must strongly caution the reader to regard these merely as tendencies I have noticed, not as definitive or inflexible rules. Each patient is different. No practitioner can pretend to understand all of human behavior. None of us knows precisely which nerve centers govern a particular behavior.

If a practitioner states to me that stomach pain, for example, always reflects a conflict with the "social self," I regard this statement as showing complete lack of respect for patients' individuality, and lack of understanding of basic osteopathic principles.

The emotional correlations I will mention from time to time are not based on any published articles or textbooks, nor on the clinical observations of others. They are simply what I have observed in my own professional experience. Interestingly, some organs (e.g. gallbladder, intestines) are relatively easy to "understand." Others (e.g. spleen) remain a mystery to me in this context.

Clinical usefulness of emotional thermal zones

These zones can be helpful in understanding the patient's problem and designing effective treatment.

Consider a male patient who presents with moderate back pain and a zone of intense pain around T6. MTD reveals a gastric emotional thermal projection. Chances are good that this patient is experiencing some significant social or professional conflict. Manipulation of the vertebrae is of secondary importance in this case. The patient is more likely to be helped by relaxation techniques, visceral manipulation, and other treatments aimed at the underlying problem, not just the somatization.

Types of emotional conflict

These are numerous. They range from mild vexation related to a minor event to high anxiety without apparent cause. The organs affected are linked to nerve plexuses, which are in turn linked to cerebral centers, often in the frontal and parietal areas.

In simple somatization, a specific organ reacts to signals from the brain in response to emotional input. Other emotional reactions are more complex, involving various parts of the body together with the cerebral centers.

There appears to be a "visceral hierarchy" related to degree of emotional conflict. For example, the gallbladder is more likely to react to minor conflicts, the pancreas to greater emotional upheavals.

Correlation between thermal intensity and severity of lesion

I am often asked, "Does a strong thermal projection indicate a severe lesion?" The answer is unequivocally no. MTD cannot be used to characterize the severity of a lesion!

Thermal intensity may be much greater for a minor gastric inflammation than for a gastric cancer. If you use MTD, it is absolutely necessary to be aware of its limitations. MTD gives us information on location, size, and intensity of a lesion, but not its severity.

If you have any reason to suspect a severe condition such as cancer, you must immediately refer the patient to an appropriate specialist.

General methodology for MTD

Communication with patient

Before performing MTD, you should give the patient some background explanation, in simple terms. Try to convey the following points:

- Problems of the body are expressed by slight thermal variations which the hand is capable of sensing and analyzing.
- Many controlled experiments have confirmed both the variations of thermal flow and the thermosensitivity of the hand.
- There is nothing magical or mysterious about MTD. To discourage this possible misconception, keep emphasizing the fact that the body emits heat at the site of a problem, and the hand is sensitive enough to detect this heat.

Some patients, as they watch you pass your hand over their body, may express the idea that you possess some exceptional or extraordinary ability or gift. This is gratifying to hear, but you must resist the temptation to agree with or reinforce this idea, which is detrimental to a proper practitioner-patient relationship. Instead, say that the only "gift" is the opportunity to develop your sensitivity and learn to perceive and analyze thermal differences of the body.

While maintaining a certain skepticism (as they should!), most patients learn to appreciate and respect MTD, especially when they realize the correctness of the conclusions given. For example, if a patient has previously been treated for a duodenal ulcer, and you recognize and comment on this fact, the patient's confidence in MTD will increase.

Nonetheless, always remain modest and prudent in your interpretation of perceived thermal flow. Our understanding is small in comparison to all that we would like to know.

Encourage the patient (especially if he seems overly impressionable) to accept whatever you tell him with some reservation. MTD is a highly subjective technique. The hand is not good at gauging absolute temperatures, despite its ability to locate and sense small differences in heat intensity.

As you learn to concentrate on hyperthermic zones, you will become increasingly adept at sensing heat. After sufficient experience, you will not be in doubt about your perception and location of thermal projections. However, do not be dogmatic or insistent about your analysis of its significance.

In MTD, thermal perception is far more reliable than its interpretation.

Dress and position of patient

The presence of clothing does not preclude MTD. Infrared waves pass through cotton and other light fabrics. However, clothing hinders precision and interpretation of thermal perception. Also, tight clothing may produce local excesses of heat. Ideally, the patient should remove as much clothing as possible prior to MTD—but respect the patient's modesty. In France, patients are less inhibited about undressing than in certain other countries.

Ask the undressed patient to lie upon the exam table for a short time before testing. In a 22°C room, five minutes should be sufficient. Arms and legs should be extended loosely, with muscles relaxed. Do not touch the patient's skin prior to MTD; this can alter Ts.

Position of practitioner

It is preferable to consistently stand on the same side of every patient. This will make anatomical markers clearer and more obvious. In general, a right-handed practitioner should position himself on the right side of the patient, and vice versa. Of course, exceptions do occur. Find out what position works best for you.

What your hand detects

The human nervous system is better at sensing changes than absolutes. Your hand cannot tell you the absolute temperature of a nearby object. But it can very reliably detect variations or changes in temperature.

Objective experiments as described earlier in this chapter have shown conclusively that the hand perceives both hypothermic and hyperthermic zones as being hyperthermic. Around 70 percent of temperature variation on the human body is hyperthermic. Don't waste time or confuse yourself trying to distinguish "hot" from "cold" zones. Simply search for temperature variations, which you will always perceive as heat excess. The important thing is the location and intensity of these thermal projections.

Sequence of perception

Thermal detection must always precede diagnosis. As you begin, do not let your mind wander through complex intellectual pathways. Have only one idea in mind: the search for zones of temperature variation! When you find one, you may be tempted to immediately attach some interpretation to it. Resist this temptation, and continue your search. Too much thinking will interfere with your ability to perceive. Diagnosis comes later.

Shapes of thermal projections

As you encounter hyperthermic zones, characterize their shapes as linear, punctiform, band-like, circular, etc., according to the scheme shown in Illustration 6-1. This system will give you clues as to whether the problem is structural or functional, and its size.

Thermal intensity

You can assess how much heat is being given off by the structure in question. Always remember that thermal intensity has no correlation with the severity of the problem. Great thermal intensity over the gallbladder simply tells us that there is a problem, nothing more. It might be simple cholecystitis, a gall stone, or a tumor.

Diagnosis: General considerations

Only after all the preceding steps have taken place can you formulate a diagnosis based on the thermal projections you have perceived.

"Prediagnosis"

Most practitioners have a tendency to "find" the same types of pathology over and over again. This tendency may be due to particular interest in a certain category of pathology, or to simple projection. When a practitioner who suffers from insomnia does a history on a new patient, one of the first questions he asks is, "Do you sleep well?"

Avoid any preconceived ideas. Don't allow the patient to draw your attention to any particular area. Don't "expect" to find hyperthermic zones in any particular area. Just let your sensing hand travel over the patient and listen to what it tells you. If you can remain objective, your hand is a highly accurate and reliable tool for detecting thermal variations, as revealed in our experiments using mechanical detectors for verification.

Memory of the body

Readers of my previous books are familiar with my favorite quotation (from the American osteopath, Rollin Becker): "Only the tissues know." All pathologies of the body, past and present, are inscribed in the tissues. This inscription is often expressed thermally.

A tubercular lesion, even when completely healed and scarred over, leaves a thermal projection. I have verified this for primary infections that occurred 30 years prior my exam. The patient may have no conscious memory of the original pathology, but the body remembers. In other words, the information we obtain from thermal projections is more reliable than verbal information from the patient.

Psychological effect on thermal projections

The power of suggestion is remarkable. A healthy patient who is verbally persuaded that he has a particular problem (e.g. intestinal spasms) may begin exhibiting physical symptoms of that problem.

Can thermal projections be created through the power of suggestion?

Talk to a patient suffering from a functional intestinal problem about his stomach. Tell him that there is certainly a hiatal hernia, mucosal inflammation, etc., and describe in detail the corresponding symptoms. Use a remote thermal detector to compare thermal projections before and after your remarks. The patient will not have a new thermal projection over his stomach, but that over his intestine may be increased, sometimes up to 1°C!

I have performed experiments of this type hundreds of times. As a general rule, a hyperthermic zone can be accentuated by psychological suggestion, but its location does not change.

Placebo effect

In many areas of medicine, the placebo effect is very real. A patient is given some medication or treatment which should in theory have no effect on his condition, and yet the condition improves. Can thermal projections be affected in this way?

I have performed many experiments using "placebo" manipulative techniques. In the case of functional problems, placebo treatment can diminish the thermal projection but never make it disappear. With structural problems, the effect of placebo treatment is negligible.

The patient's self-diagnosis

The patient may believe she already knows what the problem is. She may openly or subtly direct you to a certain part of the body, or try to convince you of the existence of a problem. This is to be avoided. Ask the patient not to talk to you at all nor use "body language" to influence you while you are performing MTD.

My suggestion: tell the patient beforehand that when some part of the body has a problem, it is expressed in a manually perceptible zone of heat. You will use your hand to feel for these zones. Afterward, you will discuss your impressions and compare them with her subjective symptoms.

In this way, the patient is not unduly frustrated about not being allowed to speak during the exam. She is interested because you are going to discover something, and content to compare her diagnosis with yours afterward. This is reinforced when she sees that the conclusions from MTD are consistent to some extent with her own opinion.

Practical methodology

USE THE PALM

Sensitivity to heat is usually greatest at the thenar eminence (Illustration 6-2, no. 1), but in some people the hypothenar eminence (no. 2) or some other part of the palm (no. 3) may be more sensitive.

The part of the palm most sensitive to heat variation generally coincides with the part most sensitive to faint mechanical stimuli. This fact is useful. Slide the fingers of your opposite hand over the palm of your dominant hand. The place where you are most aware of this mechanical pressure is usually the most thermosensitive area.

Another method is to place your palms facing each other at a distance of 4cm. The thermosensitive area will almost immediately sense the heat emanating from the other hand.

Anterior surfaces of the fingers are highly sensitive to heat, but they are not suitable for MTD because of their small size, curvature, and the

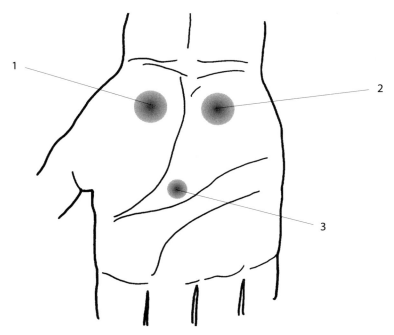

Illustration 6-2: Common Palmar Thermosensitive Zones

spaces ("cold zones") between them. The multiplicity of separated heat-sensitive surfaces on the fingers interferes with good overall thermal perception. The palm is more suitable.

Use the dominant hand

Thermal information from the sensing hand is transmitted to the brain. There is more cortical area devoted to processing information from the dominant hand compared to the non-dominant hand. If you are right-handed, use the right hand for MTD, and vice versa.

Keep the hand and wrist supple

Your shoulder, arm, forearm, wrist, and fingers must be relaxed and in a natural position. Keep your fingers supple, barely in contact with each other, not tightly pressed together. Your wrist should be very slightly extended.

Hand placement

Your palm should be roughly 10cm from the plane of the patient's skin (Illustration 6-3). Experiments have shown this is the optimal distance for sensing thermal flow.

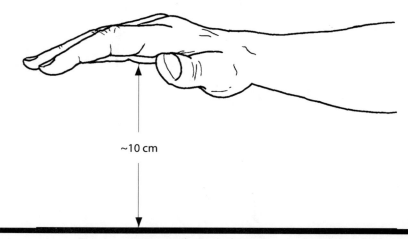

Illustration 6-3: Position and Distance of Hand

To find your ideal distance, start with your palm nearly touching the patient's skin. Move your hand perpendicularly away and stop where the greatest heat is perceived. Go slightly beyond this distance and then come back. You will have an impression of slight resistance, like a cushion of warm air beneath your palm. This is a means of sensing the intensity of thermal flow.

Follow the contours of the body

Your palm should maintain its ideal distance while also remaining parallel to the plane of the skin. Thus, as the body curves, the orientation of your hand will change.

The most thermosensitive area of the palm must remain over the plane of the skin being inspected, as though it were attached by a perpendicular thread. This is necessary in order to receive maximal information on thermal flow.

With the neck, for example, the hand remains parallel to the plane of the skin, tilting as it passes over the various elements of the neck (Illustration 6-4).

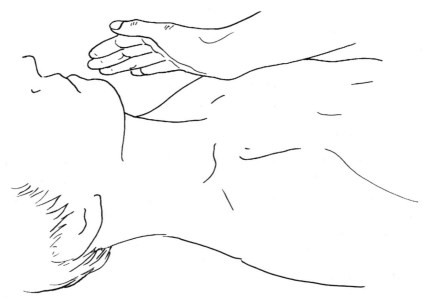

Illustration 6-4: Position of Hand for MTD over Neck

Scanning

Your sensing hand must be in continual motion. If you leave it motionless for long, you will begin detecting your own reflected infrared waves. Also, your hand will be gradually heated up by its isometric muscular work and decreased lymphatic and venous drainage.

Start with a global scan for thermal projections. Start from the head and move gradually toward the feet, exploring every part of the body in between. Many of us have a tendency to concentrate on certain parts of the body and neglect others. It is therefore helpful to have a plan for thorough scanning. One example follows; feel free to modify it.

Plan for global scanning
Anterior
- head, face, neck
- thorax, shoulders, arms, hands
- abdomen, legs, feet

Posterior
- head, neck, arms
- vertebral column, thorax, lumbar area
- pelvis, legs

Lateral
- thorax. It is not necessary to do lateral scanning of other parts of the body. The lateral thorax is of interest especially in regard to problems of the spleen or lungs.

Local scanning

As in all forms of osteopathy, we proceed from the general to the specific. After global scanning has been completed, return to the zones which appeared hyperthermic to you, and analyze them in more detail. Local scanning allows you to determine shape and density of thermal projections.

Typically, you will find three or four hyperthermic zones on a patient. For the abdomen, it is quite rare to have more than three zones. If the number of zones you have perceived is too high, clear your mind of all preconceptions and start your global scanning over again from the beginning, listening only to what your hand tells you.

CHAPTER 7

Cranium, Face, and Neck

WE BEGIN our exploration of manual thermal diagnosis with the head and neck. These are the most accessible parts of the body, and among the major focuses of osteopathy. Because there are many curves in the head and neck region, it is important to always keep your hand parallel to the surface when palpating for thermal projections over this part of the body.

Cranium

The cranium as a whole (Illustration 7-1) can be tested in the seated position. The vertex and anterior cranium can be evaluated with the patient supine.

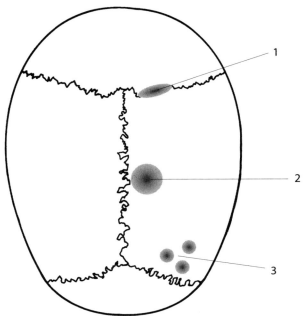

Illustration 7-1: Vertex

Sutures

Sutures give thin, linear thermal projections directly over themselves (Illustration 7-1, no. 1). It is very rare to feel an entire suture. The projections are usually ~1–2cm long. Projections are found in newborns or young children after fetal malposition and/or difficult delivery. In adults, they are found after cranial or craniofacial trauma.

The most intense thermal projection is typically over a part of the coronal suture. Such projections disappear rapidly after correction.

Cranial contents

These thermal projection are often circular zones, whose size may provide a clue to the problem. Projections over the skull are relatively easy to feel. Possibly the bones filter out insignificant "background" heat and make the projections more conspicuous.

Small circular zones

Small circular zones 1–3cm in diameter (no. 2) often reflect abnormal tissue density. A follow-up neurological exam and imaging studies are strongly suggested. In six cases I have been the first to discover tumors in this region, although some of the patients had CT scans shortly beforehand. In these cases, the projections felt very intense, as if slightly pushing my palm away from the head.

Punctiform zones

Small punctiform zones in the same part of the cranium (no. 3), can indicate a disseminated problem of brain tissue. I have felt them in patients presenting with such problems as multiple sclerosis, epilepsy, and Parkinson's disease. Often in these situations there is also a projection over T9.

Be very cautious in interpreting these small projections. The functioning of the brain is complex, and there is much we do not understand.

Large circular zones

Circular zones 3–4cm in diameter may be felt behind the eyes or superolateral to the ears, and are associated with functional disorders of vision or hearing. Larger zones (4–6cm) are most often found at the level of the right parietal and can overflow to the right frontal. They have an emotional connection which will be discussed later.

Band-like zones

These are most often found at the occipital and parietal levels after head trauma or as sequelae of meningitis. They can also indicate abnormal tension of the dural membranes.

POSTERIOR CRANIUM

You can test this with the patient seated or prone. When a patient moves from supine to prone position, the occipital region may be heated from contact with the table or cushion. Wait a few minutes before testing it.

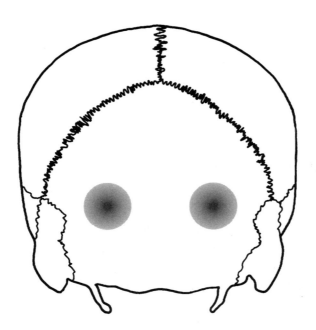

Illustration 7-2: Posterior Cranium: Circular Thermal Projections

Linear zones

These are found laterally over the lambdoid and occipitomastoid sutures. They may reflect cranial trauma (in adults) or in utero fetal constraint.

Circular zones

These are found on the left and right occipital squama and are 4–5cm in diameter (Illustration 7-2). They may relate to vision, hearing, or basilar (cerebellar) circulation.

- Vision: A circular zone in this region, when associated with a frontal zone behind the eyes (see above), indicates a functional visual disturbance (e.g. poor accommodation, poor coordination, strabismus).

- Hearing: You will also feel a temporo-occipital projection on the side of the ear concerned, most noticeable on either side of the occipitomastoid suture.

- Basilar circulation: An occipital circular zone, unilateral or bilateral, less intense and more blurry than the preceding types, is sometimes found after cervical traumas such as "rabbit punches" or thoracic outlet problems. It reflects decreased basilar circulation, particularly of the vertebrobasilar arteries, which can lead to nausea, dizziness, loss of balance, and tinnitus.

LATERAL CRANIUM

Sutures

Linear projections may be found over the numerous sutures in this area, e.g. sphenofrontal (Illustration 7-3, no. 1), sphenosquamosal (no. 2), squamosal (no. 3) and occipitomastoid (no. 4). They most often result from fetal malposition or aggressive obstetrical maneuvers.

Temporomandibular joint

A projection from the TMJ is circular, with a diameter of 1–1.5cm (no.

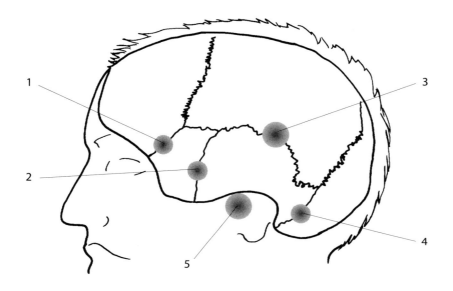

Illustration 7-3: Lateral Cranium

5). It may signify hyperactivity of this joint with irritation and inflammation of the muscles, meniscus, and/or capsule. Alternatively, it may be secondary to a problem above or below. Irritation in the TMJ area is sometimes a sign of a myocardial infarction.

MTD is a good way to check for proper bite. When there is a problem with the bite there is always hyperthermia over one TMJ or both. I have examined many patients with TMJ dysfunctions using a handheld thermal recorder, and found that the involved TMJ is always hotter. If one of these patients is given an object to bite on for 1–2 minutes, there is an increase of ~1°C in the thermal projection over the TMJ.

Temporal region

Projections here indicate problems of the ear. Otitis media causes significant thermal projection, sometimes for long periods after it has healed.

Face

Frontal region

Projections here often have emotional connections which will be described later.

Sutures

Linear zones may be found over the frontonasal and frontomaxillary sutures (Illustration 7-4, no. 1). You will almost always find them after a craniofacial trauma, motor vehicle accident, or direct impact to the face. A fracture of the nose, even an old one, always leaves a frontonasal thermal trace. The patient may have forgotten the trauma, but the "tissues remember."

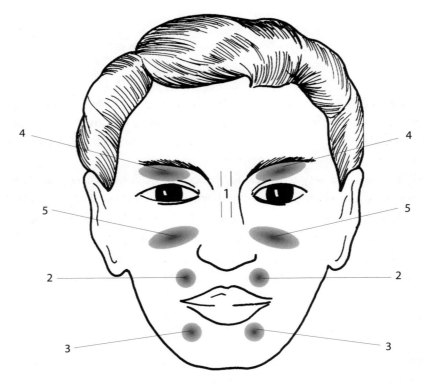

Illustration 7-4: Face

You may occasionally find projections over the zygomaticomaxillary and frontozygomatic sutures.

Jaws and teeth

The TMJ was discussed above. Projections over the maxilla (no. 2) are also of interest. A small circular zone (0.5cm diameter) here relates to the joint of a tooth in its socket. Problems with teeth sometimes have distant repercussions. I have heard cases of sciatic pain that disappears, for no logical reason, following dental work!

Small projections of vascular origin are sometimes observed over the mental foramina (no. 3). These have no pathological significance.

Parotid gland

The circular projection resulting from problems here is somewhat larger than the TMJ projection, which is located slightly posterosuperior. It reflects parotiditis or calculus in the gland duct.

Sinuses

Sinuses (especially the frontal and maxillary) are easy to feel by MTD. Also, the patient usually knows which sinus is the most sensitive or painful, and may have had x-rays taken previously. If there is a projection over a frontal sinus, you will typically feel heat over the ipsilateral maxillary sinus as well.

Hyperthermia here indicates sinusitis. When you find this, evaluate the liver. If there is a liver projection as well, the sinusitis is probably of metabolic or allergic origin. In the latter case, especially for children, reduction or elimination of dairy products and sugar from the diet may be helpful.

Frontal sinuses: Their projections, band-like and ~2cm long, are located above the orbital cavities (no. 4).

Maxillary sinuses: Their projections, roughly circular and 2cm in diameter, are found lateral to the nasal fossa and below the orbital cavities (no. 5).

Eyes

The significance of projections here depends on precise location.

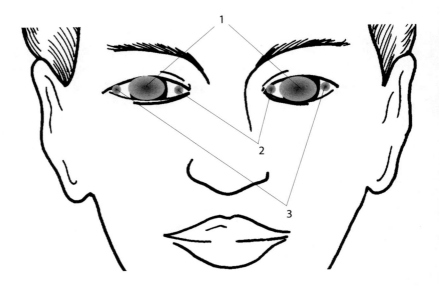

Illustration 7-5: Eyes

Bilateral projections: If the projections are centered over the irises (Illustration 7-5, no. 1), they may reflect a metabolic problem involving the kidneys, including excess uric acid production and arterial hypertension. These patients often have episodes of sharp lower back pain, especially during hot weather when the kidneys are overworked. Instruct them to decrease their consumption of animal protein. Another possible cause is ocular hypertension.

If the bilateral projections are off-center (either medial or lateral), they may reflect poor muscular coordination of the eyes.

Unilateral projection: A medial (no. 2) or lateral (no. 3) projection most often reflects a strabismus, which may not be apparent. A unilateral superior or inferior projection, if sufficiently precise and intense, is often associated with restrictions of both the cervical spine and the ipsilateral orbital musculature and fascia.

Emotional connections of the cranium and forehead

Projections in the frontal and parietal areas are often related to emotions. In fact, it is unusual to find a patient lacking such projections. Be very cautious in interpreting or "treating" them. Human emotion is a complex subject. The more information you can gather about the patient, the better.

Left frontal emotional zone

This zone (Illustration 7-6, no. 1) is 4–5cm in diameter. It has vague boundaries but feels intense. This is the center of the "relational self."

This emotional zone seems to be a center for all the organs associated with one's relationships (family, social, professional). These organs include the gallbladder, stomach, duodenum, small intestine, and superficial cardiac plexus. For more information about the emotional, psychological, and behavioral correlations of various organs, see the descriptions of the organs in subsequent chapters, and in the Appendix.

Thermal projections of the left frontal zone are common. Strong projections detectable 10cm away are related to anxiety. Weaker projections detectable only close to the skin are found in patients who are debilitated or chronically lack energy.

Right frontal emotional zone

This is a large zone (no. 2), about the same size as its counterpart on the left. This is the center of the "deep self."

The "deep self" refers to what one really is as opposed to what one appears to be—the self that one must one day find or recover. Organs connected to the "deep self" and the right frontal zone include the liver, kidneys, pancreas, and lungs.

The two frontal emotional zones communicate. When the left zone is overloaded by many different stressors, a part of the emotional tension is transferred to the right zone. Thus, if relational problems become too intense, they can become incorporated into your roots, your "deep self." The part of the right zone that exists in and of itself is termed "innate"; the

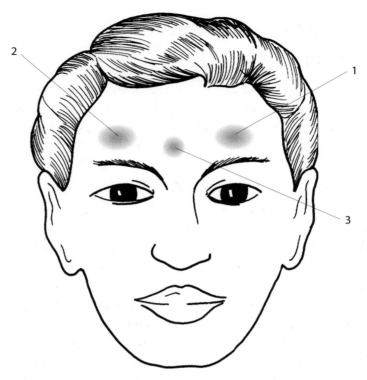

ILLUSTRATION 7-6: Frontal Emotional Zones

part which has been transferred from the left zone is termed "acquired."

Similar to the left zone, intense projection from the right zone (detectable 10cm away) can signify intense anxiety. Weaker projection detectable only close to the skin may be a sign of depression. Depending on what is going on in the patient's life, these findings may or may not be of clinical concern.

Median frontal emotional zone

This is a circular zone just above the glabella (no. 3). It is well delineated and 2–3cm in diameter. I have observed projections here in patients who are rigid or excessively "well-balanced." Such people act resolutely, following straight along their path, without asking questions. This zone does not seem to be connected to a particular organ, except possibly the intestines.

Right frontoparietal emotional zone

This is a large circular zone (5–6cm diameter) found on the right anterior parietal, near the sagittal suture (Illustration 7-7). It may slightly overflow onto the adjacent frontal, but is never near the temporal.

It is hardly ever found on the left. Frankly, I have no explanation for this fact. It is difficult to offer scientific explanations when dealing with emotions.

This is the center of the "emotional past."

All psychological or emotional events that significantly affect us are eventually inscribed in this zone. While of course this is a busy area, sometimes certain events take on special meaning, which is evident with MTD. The hippocampus, hypothalamus, and limbic system are also concerned with emotion and behavior. Are these brain structures connected to the frontoparietal zone?

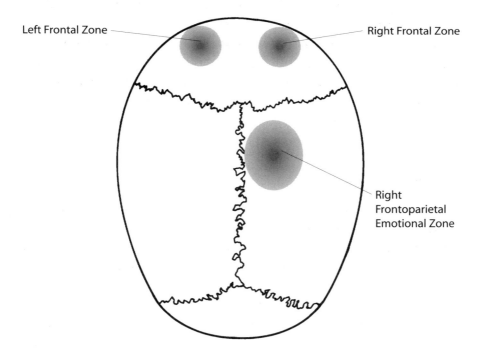

ILLUSTRATION 7-7: Right Frontoparietal Emotional Zone

Neck

The patient should be supine with neck relaxed when you perform MTD in this region. If the patient has just changed from a different position, wait a few minutes so that thermal projections can equilibrate and any moisture present can evaporate.

The thyroid gland, and large arteries and veins of the neck, radiate significant heat. In children, one frequently finds projections over the larynx in cases of recurrent sore throat. If you find heat over the larynx in an adult, check both kidneys. If you find projections over all these zones, especially in combination with recurrent lower back pain, search carefully for some infectious process.

Thyroid

The projection from this organ is either circular or a vertical band 2–3cm long. It is located to the right or left of the midline, about three finger-widths above the clavicle (Illustration 7-8, no. 1).

You can only rarely feel the isthmus. The most heat is produced by the lobes, especially the right lobe. A large, faint projection from a single lobe indicates a mild hormonal imbalance. A small, intense projection over one lobe may reflect the presence of a nodule or invasive process. Large, faint projections over both lobes indicate significant hormonal imbalance or excessive hormonal activity.

Blood vessels

Vascular problems of the neck are easy to feel by MTD. Projections from the carotid arteries are inferior and slightly medial to that of the thyroid (no. 2). The subclavian arteries are important for many reasons, including their relationship with the basilar circulation. Projections from the subclavians are small, circular, and located 1–2cm superolateral to the sternoclavicular joints (no. 3).

Projections at either of these locations may reflect vascular compression of the thoracic outlet due to pleuropulmonary problems or physical trauma. In addition, with some other pathological conditions, such as atherosclerosis, one can feel the carotids laterally on the neck. MTD will reveal short bands (~1cm long), mostly on the lower middle neck.

Pleuropulmonary problems

If you find a projection of blood vessels of the neck, look for superior thoracic pleuropulmonary projections for confirmation. These are found just under the middle of the clavicle (no. 4). See Chapter 8 for more information.

Trauma

A trauma-related thermal projection on the neck is often associated with an ipsilateral cervical or occipital problem. There may be a hemodynamic imbalance, involving the vertebral and basilar arteries, which is easily detectable by MTD. When this occurs it is almost always the subclavian and brachiocephalic arteries that give off thermal projections.

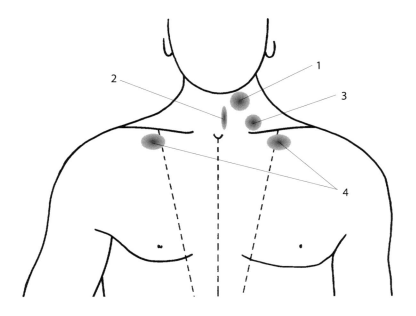

Illustration 7-8: Neck

CHAPTER 8

Thorax

FOR CONVENIENCE, I divide the thorax into superior and inferior portions. The superior thorax is bounded above by the clavicles and suprasternal notch, below on the right by the superior border of the liver (rib 5), and below on the left by the superior border of the stomach (rib 6). The inferior thorax continues from here to the inferior border of the ribcage. I will also briefly consider the "lateral thorax" at the end of this chapter.

Superior thorax

ARTICULATIONS

Clavicular joints

Hyperthermic zones over the clavicle itself are uncommon. When present, they consist of punctiform zones over the acromioclavicular and sternoclavicular joints (Illustration 8-1, no. 1). These indicate an articular problem, symptoms of which may manifest some distance away. Compensations for these problems may occur, ipsilaterally, in the cervical area, shoulders, or sternal articulations.

Adson-Wright test: If you find a projection over the sternoclavicular joint, perform the Adson-Wright (also known as Sotto-Hall) test. This consists of monitoring the radial pulse while moving the arm in abduction/ lateral rotation to 90° with the patient seated. The normal (negative) result is that the pulse does not disappear during any part of the arm movement, and its strength stays constant.

A positive Adson-Wright (i.e. the pulse disappears or becomes weaker) means that there is some tissue restriction on the ipsilateral side. The restriction may be around the cervicothoracic junction, or below the subclavian artery. If the pulse decreases when the sternoclavicular joint

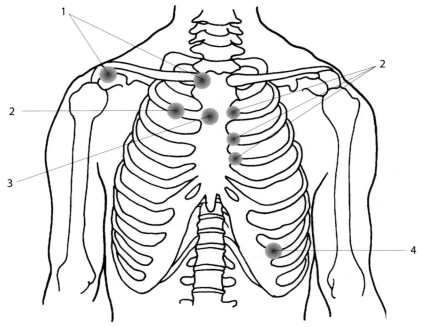

Illustration 8-1: Superior Thoracic Articulations

is compressed, the tissues around this joint are causing direct mechanical tension or an indirect reflexogenic effect on the subclavian artery.

The patient should not be supine during this test; this position relaxes a large part of the tissues capable of abolishing the pulse. For accurate readings, the patient should be sitting up during this test.

Sternocostal and costochondral joints

Problems with these joints also manifest themselves as punctiform projections (no. 2). These joints affect the subclavian vessels less often than the sternoclavicular joints.

Focus on the left fourth and fifth joints. Problems here can produce chest pain in men and pain radiating into the breast in women.

Sternomanubrial joint

This joint, located at the same level as the second sternocostal joint, gives a large, round projection (no. 3). A common cause is motor vehicle accidents in which the patient was wearing a safety belt.

Projections around the xiphoid process are usually connected with hiatal hernia. This will be discussed later.

Costal cartilage tears

Tears of the cartilage that connects the ribs to the sternum may occur during a fall directly on the side or stomach. Such tears are usually not visible on radiographs, but are quite painful and debilitating, and have adverse effects on nearby organs. A lower costal cartilage tear on the left (no. 4) will affect the stomach, gastroesophageal junction, and splenic flexure of the colon.

SUPERIOR LUNGS AND PLEURA

The body never forgets pleuropulmonary lesions. Even decades after the problem, these zones can still radiate heat. I have extensive experience with pleuropulmonary problems from working as a physiotherapist in the pulmonary service of the Centre Hospitalo-Universitaire of Grenoble before entering osteopathy. My thanks once again to Doctors Roulet and Arnaud and Professor Paramelle, who taught me so much during this period.

Pleuropulmonary problems, especially major ones, manifest as circular zones 2–3cm wide, located just below the midpoint of the clavicle (Illustration 8-2, no. 1). The location of the projection (right or left) does not necessarily indicate which side the lesion is on; it may be on the opposite side. There is a reciprocal tension imbalance of the left and right cervical attachments of the pleura. Perhaps when there is a problem on one side, the opposite (healthy) side ends up pulling more on its superior attachments during respiratory motion.

When a projection is found here, perform the Adson-Wright test. If the result is positive, ask the patient if she has dizziness, headache, or loss of balance. A pleuropulmonary restriction often leads to ipsilateral problems of the vertebrobasilar artery.

Illnesses with a strong allergic or genetic component such as asthma, eczema, psoriasis, and certain rheumatic diseases may be reflected in projections over the right bronchus, right lung, liver, and/or pan-

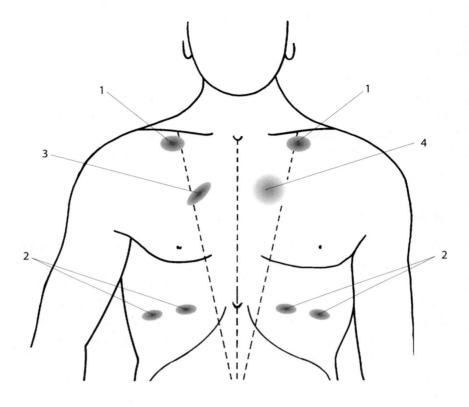

Illustration 8-2: Thorax

creas. Some genetic disorders can give a projection in the pleuropulmonary area without there being any history of lung problems. Note that some respiratory sensitivities related to infection or poor digestion are also reflected in projections over the small intestine.

Neck pain and cervicobrachial neuralgia

These types of pain are commonly found in association with restrictions of the upper pleural attachments. I have frequently seen, on autopsy, clear evidence of fibrosis of the cervical attachments of the pleura around the cervicobrachial plexus as sequelae of pleuropulmonary restrictions.

Inferior lung and pleura

It is rare to find thermal projections over the middle or inferior lung. I have occasionally observed large zones over the middle lung associated with particularly intense or active problems, or after ipsilateral lobectomy or pneumonectomy.

Pleural restrictions can result in projections at the anteroinferior border of the pleura, at the level of the rib 5 on the right and rib 6 on the left (no. 2).

Lateral lung and pleura

Some pleural restriction will give projections at the level of the costophrenic recesses, around ribs 10 and 11.

Vertebral connections

With problems of the superior lung and pleura, there are often restrictions of C7 and T1, and ribs 1 and 2. Problems of the inferior lung and pleura are associated with restrictions of T11–T12 (plus their attached ribs) and L1–L2.

Emotional connections

The pleuropulmonary region is more difficult to understand in an emotional context than organs such as the stomach and gallbladder. Pleuropulmonary restrictions or thermal projections seem to be associated with events at the beginning of life: obstetrical trauma (physical or psychological), early sicknesses, etc.

Projections over the superior pleural attachments may be emotionally related to traumas such as a "rabbit punch" (sharp blow to the back of the neck), motor vehicle accident, or fall from a considerable height. These projections are less intense and less clearly delineated than those from mechanical or infectious processes.

Bronchi

Projections of the bronchi appear as oblique bands with summits over the second and third sternocostal joints. They match the locations of

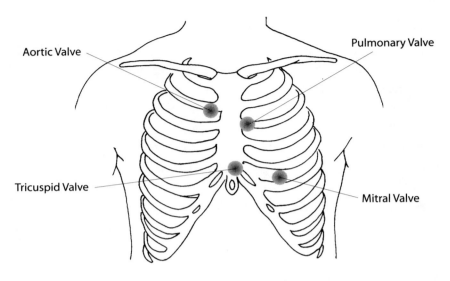

Illustration 8-3: Heart Valves

the bronchial trunks. The right trunk is more frequently felt than the left, even when both are affected (no. 3). Problems of the bronchioles are hard to detect by MTD. A projection over the right bronchial trunk in an asymptomatic person can reflect allergic tendencies.

Vertebral connection

T5 corresponds to the bronchi. It is nearly always restricted in people with asthma.

SUPERFICIAL CARDIAC PLEXUS

The projection from this plexus is circular, ~4cm wide, with vague boundaries. It is located to the left of the midline, around the second and third sternocostal and costochondral joints (no. 4).

Emotional connection

Projection over the superficial cardiac plexus can be associated with a bewildering variety of emotional states: love, kindness, passion, possessiveness, narcissism, seductiveness, jealousy, joy, exaltation, sadness, pride, arrogance, self-criticism, fear of not being recognized or liked, feeling of abandonment, etc.

HEART

The location of the heart projection is almost identical to that of the superficial cardiac plexus, but the boundaries are more distinct and intensity is greater.

Valves

Problems with heart valves produce small circular projections which are easily confused with those from costochondral joints. They are typically found over ribs 2, 3, 5, and 6 (Illustration 8-3).

Coronary arteries

Projections from these arteries are narrow vertical or oblique bands over areas of narrowing or inflammation. Even in the presence of cardiac catheterization, bands will be observed only over one or a few portions of the artery.

The right coronary artery produces an oblique band along the right sternal border, extending from rib 2 to rib 4 (Illustration 8-4, no. 1). You can generally feel only the superior part of this artery.

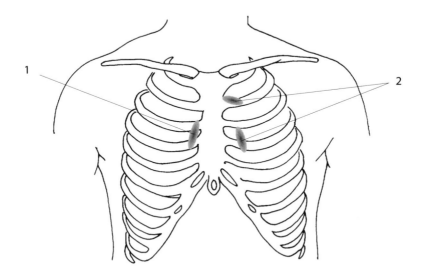

Illustration 8-4: Coronary Arteries

The projection of the left coronary artery follows the path of its anterior interventricular branch. It is a vertical band starting at rib 2 about 2cm to the left of the sternal border and running downward for 5–6cm (no. 2). In some cases you may also feel a smaller horizontal band near left sternocostal joint 2, superior to the one just described (no. 2). This superior band may give off the most heat.

Vertebral connections

Heart problems are associated primarily with restrictions of T4 and its left rib, and to a lesser extent with C4–C6 and left rib 1.

Breasts

Areolae

Thermal projections here usually reflect hormonal activity related to the menstrual cycle or breast congestion. There is a large circular zone ~3cm wide. It is rare for this zone to be displaced from the areolar center.

Zones over both areolae (Illustration 8-5, no. 1) reflect intense hormonal activity linked to the menstrual cycle. This is common in "hyperestrogenic" women, whose breasts require careful surveillance for cysts and cancer, and who tend to have cervicothoracic problems and skin ailments. Emotionally, zones over both areolae are associated with strong protective and maternal instincts.

A zone over just one areola (no. 2) may indicate inflammation or congestion of the ipsilateral breast, or a mild hormonal imbalance. In this situation, look for a projection over the ipsilateral ovary (see Chapter 10).

Breast outside areola

Small circular zones on the breast away from the areola (no. 3) are cause for concern. They indicate an area of increased tissue density.

Armpit

Two kinds of projection are encountered over the armpit (axillary fossa) (no. 4). A large projection is normal; it merely reflects the natur-

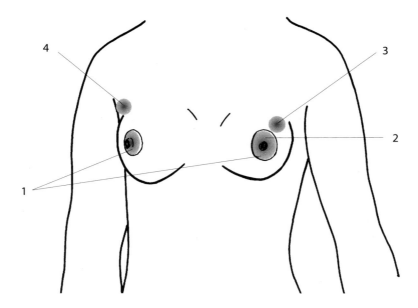

Illustration 8-5: Breasts

al hyperthermia of two body surfaces in contact. A smaller, intense, sharply delineated zone (often directed toward the superior breast) may indicate abnormal activity of the axillary lymph nodes.

Vertebral connections

Ipsilateral lower cervical restrictions often accompany (and sometimes precede) breast problems. The cervical dysfunction appears without precipitating trauma or joint disease. To a lesser extent, breast problems are associated with ipsilateral restrictions of T3–T5 and their ribs.

Emotional connections

Emotional zones on the breast are often found in women who feel strong attachment to family members or other people, or are overly protective of themselves or others. There is a sense of being "fused" with others. Emotional zones can also be related to sadness, mourning, break-up of a relationship, etc.

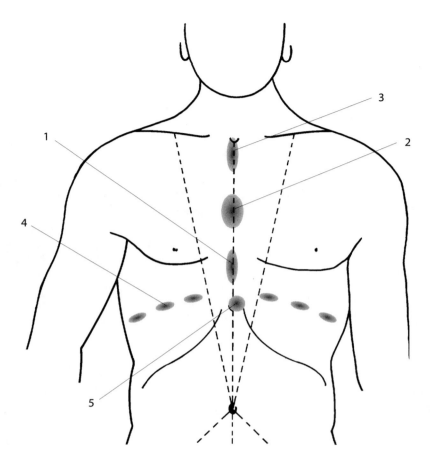

Illustration 8-6
Inferior and Central Thorax

Esophagus

The projection of this organ is a narrow vertical band ~2cm long (Illustration 8-6, no. 1), usually found over just one portion of the esophagus. Presence of this band in combination with a circular zone over the xiphoid suggests a hiatal hernia.

Vertebral connections

Problems of the esophagus are linked to restrictions of a long stretch of the thoracic spine (T4–T11).

Mediastinum and thymus

Pathologies of these structures are rarely seen, especially in an osteopathic practice. I have seen a few in hospitals and clinics, but not enough to support any generalizations.

My tentative impression is that the mediastinum has a projection over the mid-sternum, possibly radiating left or right in the direction of a bronchus (no. 2), while the projection of the thymus is higher on the sternum, possibly near the suprasternal notch (no. 3).

Inferior thorax

I consider this region to be bounded above by rib 5 on the right and rib 6 on the left, and below by the bottom of the ribcage.

Diaphragm

You rarely see a projection of the entire diaphragm. You may find a series of thin horizontal bands (2–5cm long) above the liver or stomach (no. 4). These are easily confused with costochondral zones.

Diaphragm projections can result from spasms and strains in patients with respiratory disorders. In combination with a projection over the psoas, they may indicate muscular hypercontractility. In women, in combination with a projection of the small intestine, they may reflect a tendency toward spasmophilia.

Gastroesophageal junction

Problems here give a circular projection ~3–4cm wide, with distinct boundaries, over the xiphoid process or slightly to the left (no. 5). Projections from hiatal hernias are more intense, with some radiation in a superior direction, and are usually associated with a zone over T11.

Gallbladder

This organ has a circular projection ~2cm wide with clear boundaries. It is located over rib 9 or 10, where the right midclavicular-umbilical

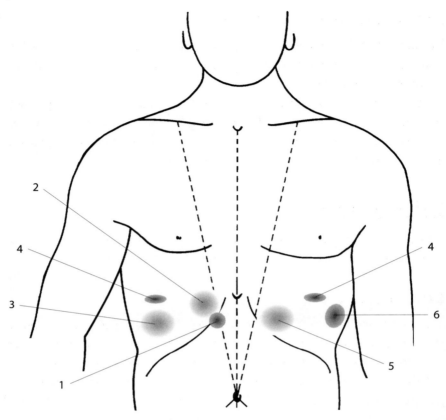

Illustration 8-7: Inferior Thorax

line intersects the lower costal margin (Illustration 8-7, no. 1).

Extension of this projection superiorly or inferiorly suggests a problem of, respectively, intrahepatic biliary function or the common bile duct. Gallstones only produce projections if their presence irritates the lining of the gallbladder.

Projections over both the gallbladder and areola suggest a hormonal imbalance, e.g. excess estrogen. The patient usually has premenstrual digestive problems that improve abruptly when menstruation begins.

Vertebral connections

Gallbladder problems are associated with restrictions of C4–C5 on the left and T7–T9 on the right. The laterality is typical of acute attacks; the restriction can become bilateral over time. Intense pain at the inferior angle of the right scapula is perceived by some with gallbladder pathologies.

Emotional connections

The gallbladder reacts to minor aggravations affecting the "superficial self": annoyance, frustration, dissatisfaction, anxiety, or moderate stress. Emotional zones are still circular, but somewhat larger and less distinct than zones with purely physical causes.

With these emotions, the patient may feel some tension underneath the liver, between the xiphoid process and the gallbladder projection. There may be an impression of discomfort or a stitch in the side. Following the localized abdominal discomfort, there may be a migraine headache, starting on the left (including pain behind the left eyeball) and rapidly becoming generalized.

LIVER

I am continually amazed at the number of physicians who disregard the existence of functional hepatic disorders. The liver is subject to a variety of problems. Palpation of the liver by an experienced person provides considerable useful information.

Intrahepatic biliary aspect

When evacuation of bile is restricted by poor drainage and/or increased viscosity, you will observe a projection the size of the patient's palm above the gallbladder projection (no. 2). This projection is large and indistinct, and situated mostly on the right side of the right midclavicular-umbilical line. There are often elevated levels of serum cholesterol and triglycerides.

Parenchyma

Parenchymal problems (e.g. hepatitis) give an indistinct projection, larger than the palm of the hand, over the right lateral liver (no. 3).

Around 80 percent of people in France will contract type A (relatively benign) hepatitis at some point in their lives, usually without even knowing they have it.

Attachments

Attachments of dense organs can be stretched or injured by motor vehicle accidents, falls on the back, etc. When this happens to the liver, you will find a small projection over one or both triangular ligaments (no. 4). The left triangular ligament is located beneath the nipple at the level of rib 6. The right triangular ligament is located at the intersection of the axillary line and rib 5. These projections are often accompanied by right-sided restrictions of costovertebral joints 7 and 9, and C5–C6.

Hepatic flexure of colon

This projection is on the right, beneath that of the parenchyma, at the level of ribs 9 and 10. It overflows onto the abdomen in the direction of the transverse or ascending colon.

Vertebral connections

Liver problems are often associated with restrictions of T7–T9, and C5 on the right. The ribs overlying the liver may also be restricted.

Emotional connections

Major stress affecting the "deep self" is often reflected in the liver. Projection from the parenchyma typically accompanies asthenia. That is, the patient displays chronic fatigue, lack of energy, lack of enthusiasm, inability to enjoy life, and hypersensitivity to various types of stress. Not only physical energy, but also psychological and intellectual energy are affected. The patient can take care of routine daily tasks but shows little capacity to innovate or create. Conversely, psychogenic nervous depression may adversely affect the parenchyma.

The liver reacts to intense anguish, "unbearable difficulties," cyclic rage, or strong fears (whether based on reality or imagination).

Patients with liver problems can explode with uncontrollable anger and then quickly calm down. The liver is the organ of identification with one's deep self, the roots of one's personality.

Stomach

Gastric air pocket

This projection is large, with vague boundaries, situated to the left of the left midclavicular-umbilical line at the level of ribs 6 and 7 (no. 5). It rarely extends lateral to the left nipple. Causes include gastritis, ulcer, duodenitis, "nervous stomach," and appendicitis.

Phrenogastric attachments

Restrictions of these superior attachments produce a projection over the left hiatal area or the air pocket. There is usually a mechanical problem involving the gastroesophageal junction, phrenogastric ligaments, etc.

Splenic flexure of colon

This projection is circular, and smaller than that of the air pocket. It is located superolaterally to the latter, and is easily confused with it. The splenic flexure projection often overflows onto the abdomen in the direction of the descending colon.

Vertebral connections

In association with problems of the stomach, we find left-sided restrictions of T6 and rib 6. For the gastroesophageal junction, we find right-sided restrictions of T11–T12, L1, and rib 7.

Emotional connections of the stomach are described in Chapter 9.

Lateral thorax

Most of the organs of interest are more accessible from the front. However, examination of the lateral thorax by MTD can also be helpful in some situations.

Lungs

Lung projections are difficult to perceive on the lateral thorax. Pleural problems may be felt around ribs 10 and 11.

Liver

The liver parenchyma can give a thermal projection on the lateral thorax around ribs 7 and 8. This can be used to confirm the anterior zone described above.

Hepatic flexure of colon

This projection is around ribs 9 and 10, just below (and slightly smaller than) the liver parenchyma projection.

Spleen

This is by far the most difficult organ to detect by MTD, as confirmed by my own experience and experiments using the remote thermal detector. The reason is that structural or functional disorders of the spleen are quite rare. When they do exist (e.g. Hodgkin's disease), there is a clear projection. It is located laterally over ribs 8–10 on the left, overflowing 5–6cm onto the anterior thorax (no. 6). It may also extend downward toward the descending colon.

Splenic hyperthermic zones may appear following serious infections.

Vertebral and emotional connections

Splenic dysfunction is associated with left-sided costovertebral restrictions, usually of T10 and their ribs.

The spleen is difficult to differentiate from the pancreas in terms of emotional zones. See Chapter 9 regarding the pancreas.

Splenic flexure of colon

This projection is just beneath that of the spleen. It is smaller and tends to overflow downward toward the descending colon.

CHAPTER 9

Abdomen

THE NUMBER of significant thermal projections is typically higher for the abdomen than for any other region of the body. The apparent complexity of this region is somewhat deceptive; a good working knowledge of topographic anatomy makes interpretation of MTD reasonably straightforward. However, since some projections are very close to each other, it is important to learn their configurations as well as locations. For example, hyperthermia of the right parumbilical area can reflect a problem of many structures (sphincter of Oddi, duodenum, small intestine, right kidney, etc.)

In this chapter, I will describe the usual locations and configurations of projections from the various organs and structures, and give tips on how to avoid common diagnostic "traps."

Stomach

See Chapter 8 regarding the gastric air pocket.

FUNDUS

This projection is usually at the level of ribs 7–9, since the superior end of the stomach is almost never above rib 6. The projection usually extends below the inferior limit of the thorax. It is a large zone with indistinct boundaries (Illustration 9-1, no. 1), and is found with most disorders of the stomach, some disorders of other digestive organs, and with anxiety or hyperreactivity.

BODY

Two types of projection are found with problems of the gastric body:
- a large projection, about the size of the palm, on the left hypochondrium, beneath the air pocket and a few centimeters

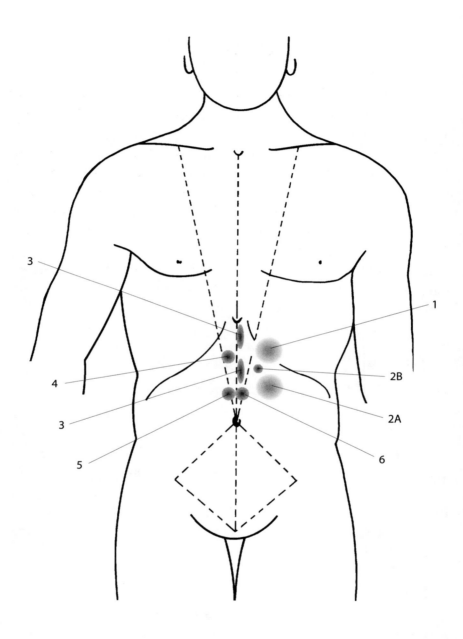

Illustration 9-1: Stomach and Duodenum

left of the midline (no. 2A). This usually relates to a non–localized problem such as spasms.
- one or a few punctiform projections in a slightly more superomedial location (no. 2B). This reflects localized inflammation or ulcers, and is often accompanied by a projection over the sphincter of Oddi.

It is possible for both these types to exist in the same patient.

Lesser curvature

This structure is located just left of the midline. Its projections are small punctiform or vertical linear zones (no. 3). It is necessary to differentiate them from other superior epigastric projections. A projection very close to the xiphoid process often reflects a hiatal hernia. In this case, the projection tends to extend into the thorax, along the midline or a bit to the right. Punctiform zones over the lesser curvature may reflect an ulcerated zone, in which case there is almost always a projection over the sphincter of Oddi as well.

Pyloric antrum

Location of this structure is highly variable. It may be at the level of the umbilicus or as far down as the pubic symphysis. Its projection is 3–4cm wide, circular with vague boundaries, and near the midline (but with similar vertical variability). When it is near the pubic symphysis, it reflects a gastric ptosis and is often accompanied by a projection over the pylorus.

Pylorus

This projection is circular and ~2cm wide, located 4 or 5 finger-widths above the umbilicus, near the midline, usually slightly to the right (no. 4). It is typically associated with ulcers of the stomach or adjacent duodenum, or with anxiety.

Vertebral connections

Left-sided restrictions of C5–C6, T6, and rib 6 are often associated with problems of the stomach.

Emotional connections

The stomach corresponds in an emotional context to the social/professional self. It represents us in relation to society and the people who surround us. This aspect is usually more important in men than women. It does not concern the real character, the deep self, the root personality. Rather it is all in us that makes up the image that we give, or want to give, to others. It can reflect desire to be recognized, creativity, pride, ambition, narcissism, hyperactivity, aggressiveness, authoritarianism, rancor, sense of social injustice, guilt, excessive or deficient self-esteem.

Trouble can arise when a person does not sufficiently differentiate his "professional personality" from his "real personality." For example, doctors need to stop being doctors when they are off duty. They should refrain from diagnosing others, giving advice, and so on.

The stomach reacts to short-term or medium-term hyperanxiety. Compared to the gallbladder, it reacts to higher levels of stress.

A good hypothetical example would be a man who sees a position of great responsibility that he thinks he deserves given to one of his colleagues. This type of professional frustration is difficult to verbalize in the confines of "polite society." Accumulation of unexpressed rancor, and a feeling of being underappreciated in relation to others, may lead initially to simple gastralgia and later to an ulcer.

The stomach, compared to other organs, reacts very rapidly to stress. I have been surprised to see cases of very young children who develop stomach ulcers from the stress of hospitalization and separation from their families. We should remember that, as author Paul Valery put it, "The child is father to the man."

In overly simplistic terms, we could say that the stomach is the organ of appearances, whereas the liver is the organ of being. This may explain why pathologies of the stomach are frequent in relatively young men at the height of their social standing, or on the "fast track" to professional success.

Duodenum

This is the proximal (first) part of the small intestine, extending from the pylorus to the jejunum.

Duodenopyloric junction

The projection of this junction is essentially the same as that of the pylorus itself (no. 4), but may project a bit more in a superior direction toward the right costal margin, slightly inferomedial to the gallbladder.

Sphincter of Oddi

This projection is on the right midclavicular-umbilical line, three finger widths above the umbilicus (no. 5). It is a small, easily detectable circular zone ~1.5cm wide.

Pancreatic or biliary problems

A projection of the sphincter of Oddi can be associated with a functional problem of the exocrine pancreas, symptoms of which are difficult to differentiate from those of the liver. This projection can also reflect problems of the extrahepatic biliary pathways, e.g., excessive bile viscosity or microlithiases.

Gastroduodenal problems

A projection over the sphincter of Oddi can also accompany gastric or duodenal ulcers. Perhaps this is due to spasm and inflammation of the sphincter.

Duodenojejunal junction

This projection is on the left midclavicular-umbilical line, three finger widths above the umbilicus (no. 6), exactly symmetrical to that of the sphincter of Oddi on the right. It is also circular and ~1.5cm wide. It can reflect problems with hyperacidity of the stomach, gastric emptying, or duodenojejunal reflux.

Do not confuse this projection with that of the left kidney, which is much larger and located slightly more superior.

Vertebral connections

Duodenal problems are often associated with restrictions of T7 and right costovertebral joint 7.

Emotional connections

These are similar to those of the stomach, tending toward more chronic or intense situation. That is to say, professional or social frustration over a short or moderate term is likely to affect the stomach. Frustration that is more intense and/or experienced over a longer term is more likely to cause problems of the duodenum.

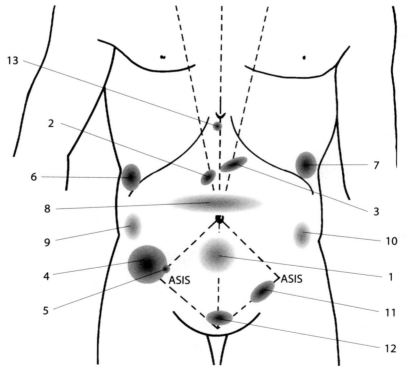

Illustration 9-2: Intestine and Pancreas

Jejunum/ileum

These are the middle and distal portions of the small intestine. Their projection is larger than the palm, diffuse, and usually located between the umbilicus and pubic symphysis (Illustration 9-2, no. 1). Its presence reflects a general functional problem of the small intestine (with associated spasm and gas), or an infection. In children, you may feel heat here following a vaccination.

There are sometimes small, distinct circular zones over this area. They signify local inflammation from causes such as torsion, ulceration, infection, or abdominal surgery. They may also be associated with spasmophilia, muscular tetany, or spastic muscular disorders.

Vertebral and emotional connections

Problems of the jejunum/ileum are associated with restrictions of T10, or less commonly T12 or L1. Emotional connections will be discussed below in combination with the large intestine.

Pancreas

The projection for the pancreas in general is an oblique band ~4–5cm long. It starts around the sphincter of Oddi projection and runs superolaterally toward the left costal margin at the level of rib 10.

Exocrine pancreas

Functional problems here give a projection concentrated around the sphincter of Oddi (no. 2).

Endocrine pancreas

This projection, which corresponds more to the body and tail of the pancreas, is closer to the costal margin (no. 3). It is associated with diabetes, various lung and skin disorders, and significant allergies.

Vertebral connections

My experience with diabetic patients shows that the most common restriction associated with the pancreas is at T9. Pancreatic dysfunction can also cause left scapular pain at the insertion of the levator scapulae.

Emotional connections

I have observed pancreatic projections linked to stress that the individual has great difficulty integrating or compensating for. Examples are violence, breakups of a relationship or family, profound injustice, death (especially violent death), sadness, depression, mourning, withdrawal, low self-esteem, lack of confidence, and paranoia. Some of these patients feel that they are under a family curse, or must suffer because their parents have suffered.

Large intestine

Cecum

This projection is a circle or band about the size of the thenar eminence. It is located above the right anterior superior iliac spine (ASIS), just lateral to the ileocecal junction (no. 4). It is associated with metabolic problems (from a bad diet, too much animal protein, or too much sugar), right lower back pain, sciatica, or right knee pain.

Ileocecal junction

This projection is circular, ~1cm wide, and has distinct boundaries. It is slightly medial or superomedial to the right anterior superior iliac spine (no. 5). It reflects hyperacidity of the ileum or improper orientation of the ileocecal junction resulting from adhesion following appendectomy or other surgery.

Appendix

The location of this structure is variable, but the most common location of the projection is McBurney's point, one third of the distance from the right ASIS to the umbilicus, and close to the ileocecal junction.

One of the pioneering studies on remote thermal detection with a machine was made by Dr. Bruno Roche, University Cantonal Hospital of Geneva, Switzerland. He examined 109 children with acute abdominal pain. Sensitivity of the thermal detector was 96 percent, and its specificity was 76 percent.

A projection in the area of the appendix does not definitely signify acute or chronic appendicitis. It may also reflect lymphadenitis or terminal ileitis. In these cases, the only subjective symptom is often sharp lower back pain plus knee pain. With lymphadenitis, there are often thermal signs that the body is having trouble organizing its defenses, e.g. projections over the liver, lung, or root of the mesentery.

Many cases of lymphadenitis occur around age 10, perhaps for immunological reasons. This is also the most common age for appendectomies—of which an estimated 40 percent are unnecessary!

Flexures of the colon

These were mentioned in Chapter 8. Their projections are partly on the inferior thorax and partly on the superior abdomen. The hepatic flexure (no. 6) is at the level of ribs 9–10. The splenic flexure (no. 7) is slightly superior (rib 8) and more lateral.

It is easy to confuse the hepatic flexure with the liver, or the splenic flexure with the gastric air pocket or spleen. A good way to differentiate these is to pay attention to the direction. For example, with the hepatic flexure, the heat goes downward past the costal margin, but this is almost never true for the liver.

Transverse colon

This is a highly mobile structure. Its projection may be felt as a band or vague circle, about the width of the palm, above the umbilicus (no. 8). It can be distinguished from the small intestine because it is not below the umbilicus, and from the stomach because it extends to the right of the midline.

Ascending and descending colon

These give vertical bands 4–5cm long on the right and left sides of the abdomen respectively (nos. 9 & 10). The bands are patchy rather than continuous. Their pathological implications are the same as for the cecum, with the possible addition of diverticulosis and polyposis.

Sigmoid colon

This projection is an oblique band 4–5cm long, on the line from the left ASIS to the pubic symphysis (no. 11). It, like the projection of the cecum, can be intense—sometimes 2–3°C higher than other organs! It may be extended in the direction of the descending colon above or the rectum below.

Hyperthermia here can reflect constipation, venous stasis, hemorrhoids, sigmoiditis, tumor, left lower back pain, or lumbosacral strains. Interestingly, a projection over the liver is almost always accompanied by one over the sigmoid, possibly because of the portal venous system that connects these two structures.

Rectum

Although the rectum is one of the hottest areas inside the body, its surface projection is not unusually intense. This zone is vaguely circular, located just above the pubic symphysis, and radiates in the direction of the sigmoid (no. 12). It is 4–5cm wide, more precise and smaller than the uterus or bladder, but bigger than the cervix or prostate. It reflects such problems as hemorrhoids and tumors. The vertebral connections of the rectum are to the sacrum and coccyx.

Vertebral connections of the large intestine

Restrictions of T12–L1–L2 are commonly associated with problems of the large intestine. The right sacroiliac joint corresponds to the ascending colon, cecum, and appendix. The left sacroiliac corresponds to the sigmoid colon and rectum.

Emotional connections of the small and large intestines

The small intestine reacts more quickly and intensely than the large intestine to emotions, but I will speak here of both together as "the intestine."

Functional problems of the intestine are more common in women; the same is probably true for emotional connections. In an emotional context, we can consider the intestine more "feminine" and the stomach more "masculine."

The intestine is the organ affected by long-term somatization, frustration, and stress. In general, shorter-term stressors impact the gallbladder and stomach, longer-term stressors impact the intestine.

"Intestinal" patients often suffer from logorrhea; they talk excessively, in a rapid, pressured fashion. This excessive talking serves to conceal their anxieties. They may speak of various illnesses, often involving the intestines. Regularity of bowel movements assumes great importance and is closely monitored.

I have observed that "intestinal" people are hyperprotective of their families. If such a woman has children, she is a mother with a capital "M." She hovers over the children, pays great attention to their bowel movements, and is obsessive in "taking care" of and supervising them. As part of a couple, the woman will dominate and protect her spouse in the same way the mother does her children. If you ask a question of the husband, the wife will answer for him.

These women may exhibit hysterical or hypochondriac behavior, making dramatic statements or gestures in regard to their problems and pains. They desire constant affection, which must be demonstrated clearly and abundantly. They are not really aware of the true needs of others. For example, the protective, dominating mother/wife may not know much about who her children and husband really are, even though she wants to be loved and recognized herself.

Celiac plexus (solar plexus)

This is the portion of the prevertebral plexus that lies on the front and sides of the aorta at the origins of the celiac trunk and superior mesenteric and renal arteries. Its projection is indistinct, ~2cm wide, and located between the xiphoid process and gallbladder (no. 13). It is often seen in agitated, upset patients.

Kidneys

Renal pathologies give intense anterior thermal projections. The kidneys are often damaged structurally by infections. They can also exhibit functional or emotionally-related problems.

Recall that the right kidney is lower than the left because of the presence of the liver.

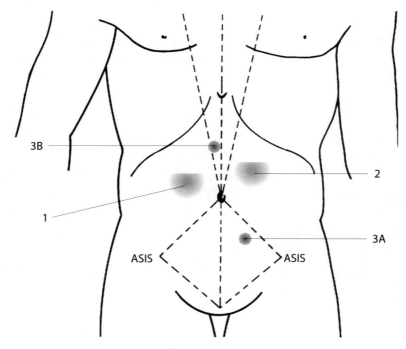

Illustration 9-3: Upper Urinary System

Right kidney

The projection is blurry and semicircular (rounded edge down), about half the size of the palm, to the right of the midline and a few centimeters above the level of the umbilicus (Illustration 9-3, no. 1). This corresponds to the inferior part of the kidney. In cases of serious infection, you may feel a projection from the superior part as well.

Right kidney projections are often associated with those from either kind of liver problem (intrahepatic biliary or parenchymal). They may also occur with ptosis. In this case, the zone is lower and extends below the umbilical level.

Left kidney

This projection, compared to the right kidney, has a similar shape and distance from the midline but is more superior (no. 2), being felt superolateral to the duodenojejunal junction. It is often associated with circulatory problems of the genitals. Recall that on the left the spermatic or ovarian vein empties into the renal vein, whereas on the right it empties into the inferior vena cava.

Bilateral kidney projections

I have observed these in association with poor general metabolism (e.g. from improper diet), hypercholesterolemia, elevated uric acid levels, muscular problems, acute or recurrent lower back pain, hypertension, and profound fatigue.

Ureter

A projection from this structure is only observed in cases of stones or ureterovesical reflux. If there is a stone in the ureter, you will feel a small but extremely intense punctiform zone, situated on the right or left side on a line parallel to the midline (no. 3A). A stone in the renal pelvis gives a projection 1–1.5cm wide, slightly lateral to the midline, 3 or 4 finger widths below the xiphoid process (no. 3B).

Ureterovesical reflux gives small circular projections inferior to a line connecting the right and left ASIS, about two finger widths lateral to the midline.

Vertebral connections

Problems with the kidneys are associated with restrictions of T7–T11 and L1–L2.

Emotional connections

The right and left kidneys have very distinct emotional implications. Bilateral kidney projections have no particular emotional significance.

Right kidney

This is the organ of frustrated intense anger. It relates to events that are "too emotional" for the liver, including deep anguish dating from early childhood. This organ can also reflect a desire to dominate along with a paradoxical fear of this desire, or other types of fear. The subject may express the fear through angry, impulsive, or out–of–control behavior.

Left kidney

This organ relates to gender, sexuality, and libido. An emotional projection here can reflect some inhibition or repression involving the genitals, not necessarily frigidity or impotence. Gender and sexuality are complex subjects. We must think in terms of their potentialities, not just their realization. A man may have no sex life and yet have the potential for one. A woman may have no children and yet have the potential to be a successful mother.

The left kidney is also affected by significant repression or inhibition of personal development. It expresses the deepest power of being. It reflects not only the life which was given to you, but also the life that you transmit. Thus, the left kidney is part of the roots of our existence. When there is a significant problem here, the subject often feels profoundly ill. Inappropriate aggressiveness, or an existential discontent or malaise, may arise from this feeling. The left kidney also reflects the fear of one's own death.

CHAPTER 10

Pelvis

WE ARE concerned here with organs of the urinary and reproductive systems. The kidneys, located in the abdomen, were described in Chapter 9.

Bladder

The thermal projection of this organ is less intense than that of the uterus (with which it is easily confused) and much less distinct that those of the ovaries and cervix. You are likely to observe it only in cases of severe cystitis, where it appears as an indistinct circle 6–8cm wide, near the pubic symphysis (Illustration 10-1, no. 1).

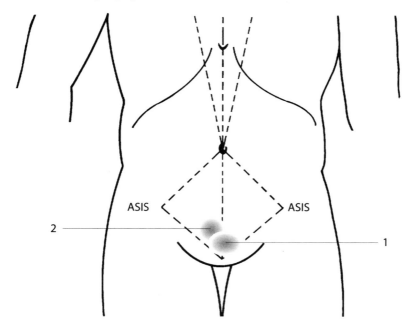

Illustration 10-1: Bladder and Uterus

Pelvis 99

Vertebral connections

Bladder problems are associated with restrictions of T11 and L3.

Uterus

It is difficult to distinguish the uterus from the bladder by MTD. Its projection is variable in location and shape, and can be up to 10cm wide. The most common location is just to the right of the midline, a bit above the pubic symphysis (no. 2). However, it can also be on or to the left of the midline, depending on the position of the uterus.

Experiments with the remote thermal detector have shown that uterine fibromas, which always feel hot by MTD, are often actually hypothermic.

At the beginning of pregnancy, you may feel a short (2–3cm) band close to the pubic symphysis. This represents the uterine cervix. As pregnancy progresses, the band disappears.

Vertebral connections

Problems of the uterus are linked with restrictions of L3–L5, sacrum, and coccyx.

Cervix

This part of the uterus has a distinct circular projection ~2cm wide, just above the pubic symphysis and left of the midline (Illustration 10-2, no. 1), the same as the prostate in men. A projection of the cervix usually signifies a mechanical problem of the uterosacral ligaments, a general pathology, or presence of an IUD.

Vertebral connections

Like the uterus, the cervix is pathologically linked to restrictions (usually left-sided) of L5, sacrum, and coccyx. The coccyx, when involved, is very sensitive to anterior mobilization.

Ovaries

These projections are well-defined circles, ~3cm wide, just below the midpoints of the lines connecting the ASISs to the pubic symphysis (no. 2). They reflect either strong hormonal activity or some abnormality. When one ovary (more often the right) is hotter than the other, it is the more active one. For example, at the time of ovulation, a projection is felt over the ovary which is releasing the egg.

A projection over one ovary not related to ovulation or high activity can result from congestion, inflammation, or tumor. Simultaneous projections over one ovary and one areola indicate a hormonal imbalance.

Projections over both ovaries during the premenstrual period indicate pelvic congestion, with associated risk of varicose veins and decreased lymphatic and venous circulation in the legs. Simultaneous intense projections over both ovaries and both areolae usually reflect strong hormonal activity, perhaps with an emotional component.

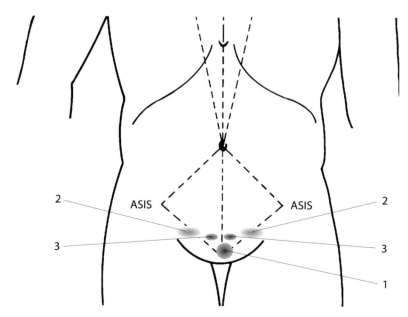

Illustration 10-2: Genital System

Vertebral connections

Problems with one ovary are often linked to ipsilateral restrictions of L3, L5, the sacroiliac joint, sciatica, or knee pain.

Bilateral ovarian problems are associated with lumbosacral joint restriction, acute lower back pain, and sciatica, especially during the premenstrual period.

Uterine tubes

These projections are either tiny punctiform zones a few millimeters wide, or small transverse bands a few millimeters wide and 1–2cm long. They are near the ovarian projections but closer to the midline (no. 3). Points indicate a mechanical problem causing poor permeability of the tubes. Bands are more likely to reflect inflammation or infection.

Vertebral connections of the tubes are not clear. They may be the same as those of the ovaries.

Vagina

This projection is quite rare. It may occur because of a tampon or vaginal infection. It is a vertical band, 2–3cm long, over the inferior part of the pubic symphysis.

Vertebral connections of the vagina are similar to those of the ovaries and uterus. With infection or inflammation of the tubes or vagina, L2 and L3 are always restricted and sensitive to palpation and mobility tests.

Prostate

This projection is identical to that of the cervix in women: a well-defined circle 2cm wide, above the pubic symphysis and slightly left of the midline (no. 1). The skewing to the left may reflect the relationship of the prostate to the left spermatic vein.

Extension of the prostate projection toward the sigmoid colon suggests a venous or lymphatic circulatory problem of the pelvis. Extension toward the ureter or left kidney suggests a genital problem or sexual dysfunction.

Simultaneous projections over the prostate and liver may reflect a sexually transmitted disease.

Vertebral connections

These are also the same as for the cervix. Men with prostate problems are also prone to left sciatica.

Seminal vesicles and testicles

Projections from the seminal vesicles are rare. They reflect an infectious problem, or sequelae from ectopic dislocation of a testicle. The location is 6–7cm below the prostate, slightly left or right of the midline.

Projections from the testicles are also quite rare, sometimes occurring with epididymitis. Pathology of a testicle may give a projection in the same place as the prostate or sigmoid colon.

Inguinal hernia

These give intense projections easily confused with those from pelvic organs. They are typically well–defined circles ~1cm wide, just above the midpoint of the line connecting the ASIS to the pubic symphysis.

Emotional connections

One might expect the pelvis to have considerable emotional connections and reactivity. Actually, I have found that there is very little, and what is there is elusive and difficult to analyze. Compared to organs of the abdomen, those of the pelvis show minimal reaction to short- or long-term emotional stimuli. Either that, or their emotional significance has escaped me. I have occasionally heard gynecologists and midwives suggest that uterine fibroids have emotional causes, e.g., that they represent the "last child" a woman would like to have.

When a person receives bad news or is at the scene of a violent assault, they commonly experience stomach cramps, gallbladder tension, intestinal or bronchial spasms, and other abdominal or thoracic symptoms. It is quite rare to hear such complaints involving any part of the pelvis. Some pelvic disorders, such as amenorrhea, may be related to long term stress, but it is difficult to believe that they are of local origin. More likely they originate from the central nervous system.

The emotional projection of the pelvis seems to correspond to the hypogastric plexus. It is a circular zone half the size of the palm, 6–7cm above the pubic symphysis, at the midline but usually overflowing to the left. This projection is often associated with that of the left kidney. The hypogastric plexus itself often reacts, in concert with the solar plexus and small intestine, to generalized heightened emotional states such as excitement, fear, infatuation, and high stress.

CHAPTER 11

Posterior Visceral Projections: Osteoarticular System

WHILE THE anterior aspect of the body is the focus of manual thermal diagnosis, this in no way releases us from the obligation to feel for thermal projections posteriorly. Not only will this yield information about the vitally important axial skeleton and other musculoskeletal structures, it also enables us to check some of the anterior findings.

For many years we have thought that the extremities, particularly the lower extremities, are too often overlooked in osteopathy. When there are knee or ankle symptoms, these structures are examined. But in the absence of local complaints, they are ignored. This chapter includes information on the thermal projections of these structures in the hope that they will be included more often in the global osteopathic gaze.

Posterior visceral projections

As mentioned before, the patient–supine position is almost always the best one for MTD. Anterior projections are so clear that it is seldom necessary to look closely at the posterior side. When I check the back, it is usually to confirm renal, hepatic, or pulmonary zones which I have felt anteriorly (see Illustrations 11-1 and 11-2).

LIVER

This posterior projection is circular, 6–7cm wide, and located lateral to the transverse processes of T7–T9, usually close to the posterior angles of the corresponding ribs. It indicates a parenchymal or intrahepatic biliary problem (see Chapter 8).

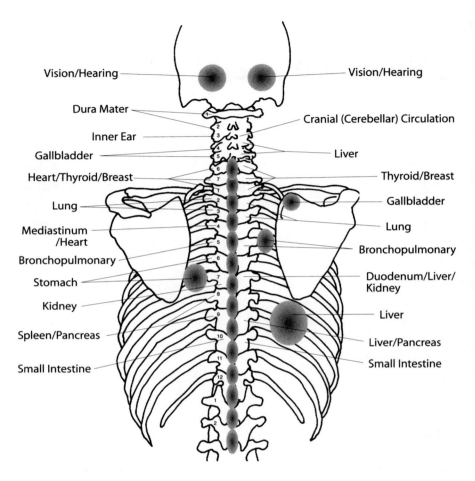

Illustration 11-1: Posterior Vertebral and Visceral Projections I

KIDNEYS

Only intense renal problems give posterior projections, which are located below the middle of rib 11, next to the transverse process of L2.

LUNGS

This zone is circular and located between the medial scapula and the transverse processes of T3–T5. Anterior projections of the lungs are very clear and I seldom use the posterior ones.

Gallbladder

This small, circular zone is located on the superomedial right scapula, over the levator scapulae insertion. This is a well-known reflex point of the gallbladder, due to a sensory branch of the phrenic nerve which also innervates the gallbladder. This posterior zone is inconsistent and less reliable than the anterior gallbladder projection.

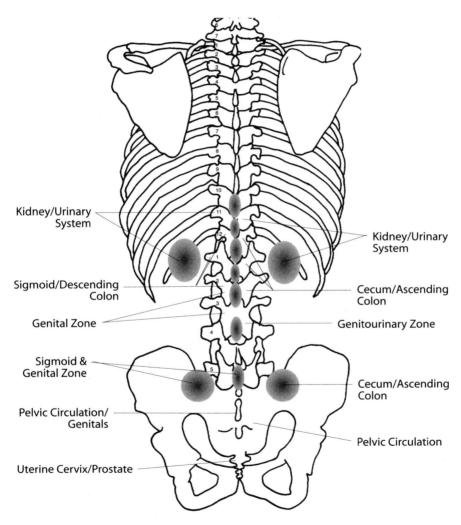

Illustration 11-2: Posterior Vertebral and Visceral Projections II

Stomach

This is a large, indistinct zone located between the medial edge of the left scapula and the transverse processes of T6–T8. Again, this posterior projection is less consistent and therefore less reliable than the anterior one.

Osteoarticular system

The bones and joints of the trunk and limbs can also give thermal projections of various sizes and shapes.

Large projections: These are typically circular and intense, and reflect problems of joints or joint capsules. The size of the projection is correlated with the size of the joint or capsule. A knee gives a much larger projection than a metatarsophalangeal joint.

Linear or band-like projections: These correspond to tendons and ligaments, and follow their anatomical course. Micro-tears and small periosteal ruptures give a linear projection associated with a punctiform zone.

Punctiform zones: These indicate very localized problems with a tendon, ligament, or meniscus. The projection is easily detected and is directly over an injury.

Fractures also give a small, intense projection.

Vertebral column

Projections from vertebrae are usually circular and 2–3cm wide. Their location is highly significant.

Spinous processes and reflexogenic zones

In my early years of practicing MTD, I thought that zones over spinous processes reflected local mechanical problems of the vertebrae. Experience showed that they often reflect visceral reflexes. My eminent colleague, Vincent Coquard, was the first to teach me about the reflexive significance of spinal projections, and the necessity of differentiating spinous processes from transverse processes. In the cervical spine, both these types of processes can give thermal projections.

The following list tells which organs are pathologically linked with projections over specific vertebrae or ribs (see Illustrations 11-1 and 11-2). This list is based on my experience with thousands of patients. Naturally, you will encounter occasional exceptions.

- C1–C2: dura mater
- C3: cerebral (especially cerebellar) circulation
- C4–C5: liver, gallbladder
- C6–C7, T1, rib 1: heart (left), thyroid, breasts
- T1–T2, ribs 1–2: lungs
- T3–T4: lung, mediastinum, heart
- T5: bronchi
- T6: stomach
- T7: duodenum, liver, kidney
- T8–T9: liver (right), pancreas, spleen (left)
- T10: small intestine
- T11–T12: kidneys, bladder
- L1–L2: small intestine, colon, pancreas
- L3–L4: genital organs
- L5, sacroiliac: cecum, sigmoid, genital organs
- sacrum, coccyx: uterus, uterine cervix, prostate

Spinal facet joints

Projections of the joints between superior and inferior articular facets are circular, 1–2cm wide, and located 2–3cm from the spinous processes. They reflect a restriction or inflammation of these joints.

Costovertebral joints

These projections are similar to those of the interapophyseal joints, and located about three finger-widths lateral to the spine, over the joints concerned.

Knee

I will describe the knee and foot joints in some detail here, from the point of view of MTD. The principles conveyed apply equally well to other peripheral joints (shoulder, wrist, etc.), which I am therefore omitting for the sake of brevity.

Any time you feel projections over the knee, determine whether they radiate in the direction of the peroneal groove or the supracondylar muscles.

After trauma to the knee there are usually lesions of muscles or ligaments that, if not treated, delay the healing process or cause decreased long-term mobility.

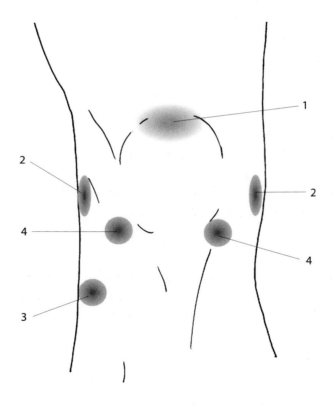

Illustration 11-3: Knee

Joint capsule

The patient is supine with legs extended. The projection of the knee joint capsule is large, starting three finger-widths above the patella and extending two finger-widths below it, to the superior part of the tibial plateau, or proximal tibiofibular joint. The superior aspect is most commonly felt (Illustration 11-3, no. 1).

In the patient–prone position, to either side of the joint, you may feel large but weak projections corresponding to popliteal cysts.

Any time you feel projections over the knee, you must also carefully examine the hip and foot.

Ligaments

The collateral ligaments are most likely to be felt by MTD. Their projections are ~2cm wide and centered over the femoral condyles (no. 2). They often extend to the superior and inferior attachments of the ligaments.

The cruciate ligaments give a projection similar to—and difficult to differentiate from—that of the joint capsule. When the knee is flexed, its anterior surface is increased. In this situation, you may be able to feel that the projection from an anterior cruciate ligament is relatively slightly medial, while those from the posterior cruciate ligaments are more posterior. However, you cannot rely on MTD alone to distinguish them.

Fibular head

A projection from the lateral collateral ligament is commonly accompanied by one from the proximal tibiofibular joint (no. 3). There may be stretching of the joint capsule or of muscle insertions around the distal attachment of the ligament.

Menisci

These can be tested in the supine position. The legs can be extended or, preferably, flexed to increase surface area of the knee. The projections of the menisci are either punctiform or small and circular, and located right or left of the patellar tendon (no. 4). Projections of the menisci are almost always accompanied by projections of one or both collateral ligaments.

Nontraumatic problems

When knee problems are unrelated to trauma or compensation for proximal or distal biomechanical problems, the cause may be a rheumatic or malignant process. Such problems produce large projections difficult to distinguish from that of the joint capsule.

Some pathologies of the kidneys or genital organs can lead, via irritation of the femoral nerve, to capsulitis with a weak thermal projection, usually on the medial side of the knee.

ANKLE AND FOOT

The patient should be supine, with hips and knees extended.

Joint capsule of ankle

This projection is large, extending from both sides and above and below the line of the joint (Illustration 11-4, no. 1). Any time you detect a problem of the ankle, always test the knee. Problems of these two joints are typically interrelated.

Ligaments

The supporting ligaments of the ankle include the deltoid ligament medially and the talofibular and calcaneofibular ligaments laterally. Their projections are bands 1–2cm wide (no. 2). The orientation of the projections helps us evaluate participation of the joint capsule or nearby tendons or muscles in problems of these ligaments.

Tendons

When evaluating problems of the ankle or foot, remember that many of the tendons come from muscles whose bodies are a considerable distance away, on the leg. Problems with leg muscles such as the extensor and peroneal groups (no. 3) can contribute to the simultaneous destabilization of the knee, ankle, and foot joints. They can also reflect a general mechanical imbalance or a visceral problem.

Bones

Each foot is comprised of 26 interdependent bones (talus, calcaneus, five anterior tarsals, five metatarsals, 14 phalanges). An ankle sprain is always accompanied by restrictions of some of the smaller distal

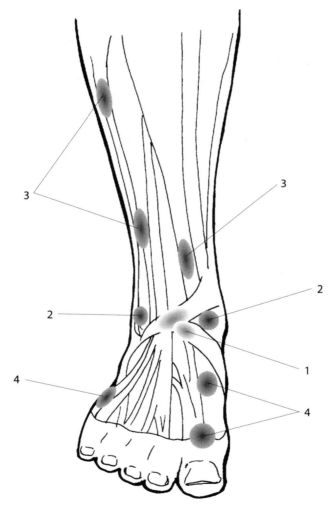

Illustration 11-4: Ankle and Foot

bones. The tendons and ligaments inserting on the small bones naturally give off projections in this and other dysfunctional situations (no. 4). Familiarize yourself with the bony anatomy of the foot and the projections found in this area. Since the foot is the "foundation" of the human osteoarticular system, problems here can have wide-ranging repercussions.

Plantar arches

MTD applied to these arches gives several types of information. First, we can look for pathology of the individual bones, joints, muscles, and tendons that comprise the arches and the plantar surface of the foot. Second, we can observe signs of poor arch support. Third, projections here may coincide with visceral reflex zones.

Plantar arch restrictions are often the outcome of or the point of origin for mechanical lesion "chains." These restrictions give clear thermal projections.

The reflexogenic zones of the plantar region are a complex and fascinating research area which I am still exploring. At this stage I can offer a couple of preliminary general impressions:

- The medial part of the plantar arch is linked more to visceral problems, the lateral part more to cranial or vertebral problems.
- The anterior part of the plantar arch is linked more to the shoulders and arms, the posterior part more to the hips and legs.

CHAPTER 12

Afterword

MTD can make an important, perhaps even indispensable, contribution to complete diagnosis of a patient. Very fine manual thermal sensitivity and perception are obviously required. However, to locate a thermal variation, even with great precision, is not enough to come up with a diagnosis. You also need rigorous knowledge and experience of topographical anatomy in order to define the areas of conflict. Only then can a reliable diagnosis be made. The illustration on the next page summarizing the main anterior thermal projections (Illustration 12-1) should only be used as a guide towards this end.

Much remains to be learned about the mechanical and thermal sensitivity of the human hand. The skin is sensitive to not only infrared but also other portions of the electromagnetic wavelength spectrum. It is toward these other wavelengths that I plan to increasingly direct my research in the future.

Working with MTD allows us to improve our perception and understanding of other sensory information. An integrated approach is essential for a manual diagnostic/therapeutic system aimed at decoding as many as possible of the messages emitted by the tissues and organs of the body.

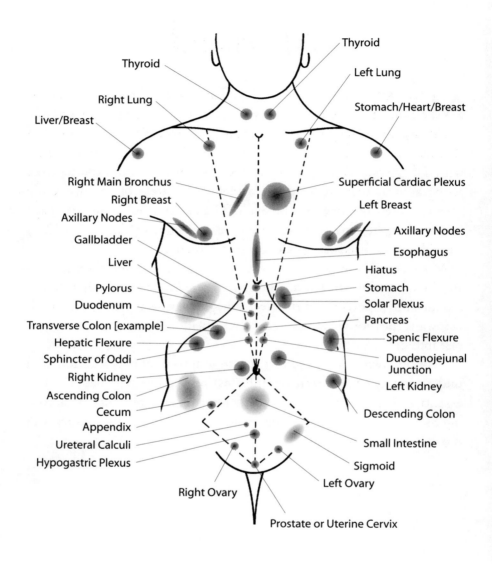

Illustration 12-1:
Summary of Main Anterior Thermal Projections

APPENDIX

Psychological, Emotional, and Behavioral Correspondences of the Organs

Stomach
Social Self/Appearances

Aggressiveness
Ambition
Anxiety
Appearances
Arrogance
Authoritarianism
Boldness
Communication
Compulsive lying
Conviction
Creativity
Culpability
Deception
Decision
Defiance
Demanding
Domination
Enthusiasm
Extroversion
Failure
Frustration
Generosity
Gratitude
Hyperactivity
Identification with others
Impatience
Insomnia
Introspection
Irritability
Jealousy
Masculinity
Megalomania
Narcissism
Obsession
Overly self-critical
Paranoia
Persecution
Pessimism
Pride
Projection
Punishment
Representativeness
Seduction

Sociability
Success
Underly self-critical

Intestines
The self

Abandonment
Anxiety
Attachment
Blaming
Censure
Complexes
Contrariness
Control
Dependence
Deprecating others
Discipline
Domination
Duplicitous
Emotional reactions
Family
Fear of decision
Fear of offending
Femininity
Frustration
Fusion
Generosity
Gratitude
Greed
Histrionism
Hyperprotection
Hypochondria

Hysteria
Inhibition
Insomnia
Irritability
Logorrhea
Mania
Meticulousness
"Motherhood"
Obsessiveness
Oedipus complex
Paradoxical reactions
Pessimism
Possessiveness
Prohibition
Protection
Punishing attitude
Repression
Ritual
Routine and rote behavior
Shame
Social status
Somatization
Stubbornness
Territoriality

Liver
Deep Self/Being

Allergies
Anguish
Arrogance
Blaming
Cyclic violence

Deep energy
Deep frustrations
Deep self
Existential fear
Identification with others
Imago
Insomnia
Intellectual energy
Introversion
Low self-esteem
Moral energy
Overly high self-esteem
Prohibition
Rage
Rancor
Rigidity
Sadness
Self-destruction
Thoughtlessness

Heart
Others

Affection
Arrogance
Attachment
Bitterness
Deception
Deprecating others
Dyspnea
Emotional hyperactivity
Excitement
Frustration

Fusion
Generosity
Hate
Jealousy
Joy
Love
Maladaption
Narcissism
Overexcitement
Overly high self-esteem
Pessimism
Pride
Repressed anger
Repression
Seduction
Self-sacrifice
Sentimentalism
Shame
Sqeamishness
Stress
Transcendence
Treason

Lungs
Inheritance

Allergies
Arrogance
Chilhood problems
Control
Generosity
Genetic memories
Genetics

Infections
Infectious memories
Overly high self-esteem
Protective attitude
Resistance (physical and moral)
Traumatic memories

Kidneys
Roots

Aggressiveness
Deep fear
Discontent
Domination
Drives
Excelling ones self
Exhaustion
Existential anguish
Generative force
Helplessness
Intense fear
Libido
Nonrealization
Obsession
Original anger
Original energy
Original self
Phobia
Repression
Sensuality
Sexuality
Traumatic memory

Spleen-Pancreas
Grief

Allergies
Breaking up
Death
Decompensation
Fear of death
Genetic memory
Insurmountable stress
Introversion
Melancholy
Memories of infections
Rancor
Roots
Sadness
Self-destruction
Victimization
Violence

Gallbladder
Aggravations

Aggravation
Anger
Anxiety
Deception
Dissatisfaction
Fear of trips
Fears
Feelings
Frustrations
Guilt

Phobia
"Punctuality"
Sadness
Scruples
Stage fright
Vexations

Breasts
Relations

Attachments
Breaking up

Children
Family focus
Grief
Guilt
Injustice
Isolation
Maternal feelings
Meticulousness
Overinvestment
Persecution
Protection
Sacrifice

Bibliography

Barral, J.-P., Ligner, B., et al. *Nouvelles techniques uro-génitales*. Paris: Cido et De Verlaque, 1993.

Barral, J.-P., Mercier, P. *Visceral Manipulation*. Seattle: Eastland Press, 1988.

Bochuberg, C. *Traitement ostéopathique des rhinites et sinusites chroniques*. Paris: Maloine, 1986.

Braunwald, E., et al. *Harrison's Principles of Internal Medicine*. New York: McGraw-Hill, 1987.

Chauffour, P., Guillot, J-M. *Le Lien mécanique ostéopathique*. Paris: Maloine, 1985.

Comroe, J.H. *Physiologie de la respiration*. Paris: Masson, 1978.

Contamin, R., Bernard, P., Ferrieux, J. *Gynécologie générale*. Paris: Vigot, 1977.

Cruveilhier, J. *Traité d'anatomie humaine*. Paris: Octave Doin, 1852.

Davenport, H.W. *Physiologie de l'appareil digestif*. Paris: Masson, 1976.

Delmas, A. *Voies et centres nerveux*. Paris: Masson, 1975.

Dousset, H. *L'examen du malade en clientèle*. Paris: Maloine, 1972.

Gabarel, B., Roques, M. *Les fasciae*. Paris: Maloine, 1985.

Grégoire, R., Oberlin, S. *Précis d'anatomie*. Paris: J-P. Baillère, 1973.

Hardy, J.D. "Physiology of Temperature Regulation," *Physiology Review* 41 (1961): 521–606.

Herman, J., Cier, J.F. *Précis de physiologie*. Paris: Masson, 1977.

Houdas, Y., Guieu, J.D. *La fonction thermique*. Villeurbanne: Simep, 1977.

Houdas, Y., Ring, E.F.J. *Human Body Temperature, Its Measurement and Regulation*. New York: Plenum, 1982.

Hugues, F. Cl. *Pathologie respiratoire*. Paris: Heures de France, 1971.

Issartel, L., Issartel, M. *L'ostéopathie exactement*. Paris: Robert Laffont, 1983.

Kahle, W., Leonhardt, H., Platzer, W. *Anatomie des viscères*. Paris: Flammarion, 1978.

Kamina, P. *Anatomie gynécologique obstétricale*. Paris: Maloine, 1984.

Korr, L. *The Neurobiologic Mechanisms in Manipulative Therapy*. New York: Plenum Press, 1978.

Laborit, H. *L'Inhibition de l'action: Biologie, physiologie, psychologie, sociologie*. Paris: Masson, 1981.

Lansac, J., Lecomte, P. *Gynécologie pour le praticien*. Villeurbanne: Simep, 1981.

Lavieille, J., Roux, H., Stanoyevitch, J.F. *Le Système vertébro-basilaire*. Marseille: Solal, 1986.

Lazorthes, G. *Le système nerveux périphérique*. Paris: Masson, 1970.

Mathieu, J.-P., Barral, J.-P., Mercier, P. *Diagnostic articulaire vertébral*. Paris: Cido et De Verlaque, 1992.
Poirier, Charpy, Nicolas. *Traite d'anatomie humaine*, Tomes I–V. Paris: Masson, 1912.
Prat, D., *Sensibilité de la main aux flux thermiques émipar l'organisme*. Personal notes, 1994.
Préfaut, C. *L'Essentiel en physiologie respiratoire*. Paris: Sauramps Médical, 1986.
Renaud, R., et al. *Les incontinences urinaires chez la femme*. Paris: Masson, 1980.
Robert, J.G., Palmer, R., Boury-Heyler, C., Cohen, J. *Précis de gynécologie*. Paris: Masson, 1974.
Roche, B. *L'ortoscan: une aide au diagnostic qui intéresse généralistes et spécialistes*. Geneva: Hôpital Cantonal Universitaire de Genève, 1994.
Roche, B., et al. Intérêt d'un thermo-détecteur à infrarouge mobile "Ortoscan" dans le diagnostic des douleurs abdominales chez l'enfant [à propos de 108 cas]. Geneva: Hôpital Cantonal Universitaire de Genève, 1994.
Roche, C., Dentant, T. *Recherches sur les flux thermiques émis par le corps*. Personal notes, 1992.
Rouvier, H. *Anatomie humaine*. Paris: Masson, 1967.
Scali, P., Warrel, D.W. *Les prolapsus vaginaux et l'incontinence urinaire chez la femme*. Paris: Masson, 1980.
Silbernagl, S., Despopoulos, A. *Physiologie*. Paris: Flammarion, 1992.
Smith, E. "Temperature Regulation: The Spinal Cord as a Site of Extra-hypothalamic Thermoregulatory Functions." *Rev. Physiology, Biochemistry, and Pharmacololgy* 71 (1974): 1–75.
Taurelle, R. *Obstétrique*. Paris: France Médical Edition, 1980.
Testut, L., Jacob, O. *Anatomie topographique*. Paris: Gaston Doin, 1927.
Thauer, R. "Thermosensitivity of the Spinal Cord." In *Physiological and Behavioral Temperature Regulation*, edited by J. D. Hardy, et al., 472–92. Springfield: C. C. Thomas, 1970.
de Tourris, H., Henrion, R., Delecour, M. *Gynécologie et obstétrique*. Paris: Masson, 1979.
Upledger, J.E., Vredevoogd, J.D. *Craniosacral Therapy*. Chicago: Eastland Press, 1983.
Waligora, H., Perlemuter, L. *Anatomie*. Paris: Masson, 1975.
West, J.B. *Physiologie respiratoire*. Paris: Medsi, 1986.
Williams, P., Warwick, R., eds. *Gray's Anatomy*. Edinburgh: Churchill Livingstone: 1980.
Wright, S. *Physiologie appliquée à la médecine*. 2d ed. Paris: Flammarion, 1974.

Index

A
Adson-Wright test, 69–70
Age, body temperature and, 13
Anger, 82, 98
Ankle, 112
Apocrine sweat glands, 35
Appendix, 92–93
Areas scanned, 54
Arms, 114
Arterial blood, 15
Ascending colon, 94

B
Bands, 42
Basilar circulation, 58
Becker, Rollin, 49
Black body, 9
Bladder, 99, 109
Blood vessels, 66
Blood, heat transfer and, 9, 14
Bloodstream, convection and, 20
Body, definition of, 8
Brain disorders, 56
Brain, temperature of, 16–17
Breasts, 76, 109
Bronchi, 73–74, 109
Bulboid corpuscles, 33

C
Cecum, 92, 109
Celiac plexus, 96
Cerebral circulation, 109
Cervix, uterine, 100, 109
Children, 61
Circadian rhythm, 13, 24
Clavicular joints, 69
Cold receptors, 30
Colon, 109
Conduction, 8, 20
Convection, 8, 20
Coquard, Vincent, 109
Core, 11. *See also* Body
Coronary arteries, 75–76
Costal cartilage tears, 71
Costochondral joints, 70
Cranial trauma, 58
Cranium, 55

D
Depression, 64, 82, 92
Descending colon, 94
Diet, improper, 97
Digestion, temperature and, 14
Duodenojejunal junction, 89–90
Duodenum, 89, 109
Dura mater, 57, 109

E
Ear, inner, 17
Eccrine sweat glands, 35
Ectotherms, 5
Electromagnetic spectrum, 9
Emissivity of skin, 10
Emotional conflicts, types of, 45
Emotional past, 65
Emotional thermal zones, 43, 63–65
Emotions and organs, 44
Emotions, temperature and, 14

Energy, definition of, 5
Esophagus, 78
Estrogen, excess of, 76, 80
Ethics, MTD and, 41
Examination, methodology, 48, 51–54

F
Foot, 113–114
Frequency, 7
Functional problems, definition of, 41

G
Gallbladder, 79–80, 107, 109
Gastric ptosis, 87
Gastroesophageal junction, 79
Gender, temperature and, 14, 24, 98
Genital organs, 109
Glomera, 21
Golgi-Mazzoni corpuscles, 34
Guieu, 15

H
Hardy, J. D., 9, 10, 32
Heart, 75, 109
Heat receptors, 30
Heat, definition of, 5
Heat, transfer of, 19
Hepatic flexure, 82, 84, 93
Hernia, inguinal, 103
Hippocrates, 1
Hips, 114
Homeothermic, 5
Hot and cold areas, 39–40
Houdas, Y., 15, 19, 22, 32
Hyperthermic regions, natural, 24
Hypochondriac behavior, 95
Hypogastric plexus, 104
Hypothalamus, 17, 32
Hypothermic areas, 40
Hysterical behavior, 95

I
Ileocecal junction, 92
Ileum, 91
Infrared, definition of, 6

J
Jejunum, 91

K
Kidneys, 62, 66, 96–97, 106, 109
Knee, 110–112
Krause's corpuscles, 29, 33

L
Lamellar corpuscles, 33
Large intestine, 92
Larynx, 66
Legs, 114
Lesions, severity of, 45
Liver, 61, 81–83, 84, 94, 98, 105, 109
Logorrhea, 95
Lungs, 84, 106, 109

M
Manual thermal diagnosis, what it does, 2–3
Mechanoreceptors, 32–33
Mediastinum, 79, 109
Meissner's corpuscles, 33
Memory, 49
Men, 14, 24, 95
Menstrual cycle, 6, 13
Merkel's cells, 33
Mesencephalon, 32
Microwaves, 22
Midbrain, 32
Migraine headache, 41, 81
Motor vehicle accidents, 70, 73

O

Obstetrical maneuvers, sequelae of, 58
Oddi, sphincter of, 89
Organ, dysfunction of, 42
Organs and Emotions, 44
Otitis media, 59
Ovaries, 101

P

Pain and thermal messages, 32
Pancreas, 91–92, 109
Parotid gland, 61
Pit vipers, 1
Placebo effect, 50
Plantar arches, 114
Pleuropulmonary problems, 71
Prostate, 102, 109
Psychosomatic problems, 43
Pyloric antrum, 87
Pylorus, 87

R

Rabbit punch, 73
Radiation, 9, 22
Rectum, 16, 94
Remote measurement of TS, 24
Ring, E.F.J., 15, 19, 22
Roche, Bruno, 1, 93
Ruffini's corpuscles, 29, 34

S

Scanning, 54
Scrotum, 16
Self,
    deep, 63, 82
    relational, 63
    social/professional, 88
    superficial, 81
Seminal vesicles, 103

Shoulders, 114
Sigmoid colon, 94, 109
Sinuses, 61
Small intestine, 109
Solar plexus, 96. See also Celiac plexus
Sotto-Hall test, 69
Sphincter-like areas, 42
Spinothalamic tract, lateral, 31–32
Spleen, 84, 109
Splenic flexure, 83, 93
Sternocostal joints, 70
Sternomanubrial joint, 70
Stomach, 16, 83, 85–88, 108, 109
Strabismus, 62
Stress, 43, 92
Structural problems, definition of, 40–41
Subclavian arteries, 66
Suggestion, thermal projections and, 49–50
Superficial cardiac plexus, 74
Sutures, 56, 60
Sweat, 21, 35–36
Sympathetic nervous system, 21

T

Tactile corpuscles, 33
Tactile menisci, 33
Teeth, 61
Temperature, regional variation of, 11
Temporomandibular joint, 58
Testicles, 103
Thalamic nuclei, 32
Thermal detectors, 39
Thermal intensity, 38–39
Thermal zones, 25. See also Zones
Thermodynamics, 7
Thermoreceptors, 29–31
Thymus, 79

Thyroid, 66, 109
Tissue conduction, 8
Transverse colon, 93
TB, definition of, 11
TS, definition of, 19
    variations in, 26
Tubes, large, 42
Tubes, small, 42
Tumors, 56

U
Ureter, 97
Uterine tubes, 102
Uterus, 109, 100

V
Vaccination, 91
Vagina, 102
Valves, heart, 75

Vasodilation, 21, 34–35
Vasomotor control, 21
Vater-Pacini corpuscles, 33
Venous blood, 15

W
Wavelength, 7
Wien's Law, 9
Wine connoisseur, 1
Women, 14, 24, 95

Z
Zones of conflict, 38, 40
Zones, large,
    with precise boundaries, 42
    without precise boundaries, 42
Zones, linear, 42
Zones, punctiform, 42
Zones, small circular, 42

Body text, headlines and subheads in this book are set in Adobe Jenson and Adobe Jenson Expert. This face is based on the classic Venetian roman typeface designed by Nicolas Jenson in 1470. Robert Slimbach designed the multiple master version for Adobe.

The body text was set in 13 point type on 15 points of lead. Footers, captions and callouts were set in Myriad. The software used to design and produce this book includes QuarkXPress 3.3.1 for the Power Mac and Font Creator.